Evaluating Preventive Care

Studies in Social Economics

SELECTED TITLES

STUDIES IN SOCIAL ECONOMICS

Louise B. Russell

Evaluating Preventive Care

Report on a Workshop

WITHDRAWN

THE BROOKINGS INSTITUTION
Washington, D.C.

Library of Congress Cataloging-in-Publication data
Russell, Louise B.
  Evaluating preventive care.

  (Studies in social economics)
  Workshop held May 8–9, 1986, and sponsored by the
Brookings Institution.
  Bibliography: p.
  Includes index.
  1. Medicine, Preventive—Cost-effectiveness—
Congresses. 2. Health behavior—Congresses.
I. Brookings Institution.   II. Title.   III. Series.
RA410.5.R87 1987   338.4′361444   87-9304
ISBN 0-8157-7626-8
ISBN 0-8157-7625-X (pbk.)

9 8 7 6 5 4 3 2 1

THE BROOKINGS INSTITUTION is an independent organization devoted to nonpartisan research, education, and publication in economics, government, foreign policy, and the social sciences generally. Its principal purposes are to aid in the development of sound public policies and to promote public understanding of issues of national importance.

The Institution was founded on December 8, 1927, to merge the activities of the Institute for Government Research, founded in 1916, the Institute of Economics, founded in 1922, and the Robert Brookings Graduate School of Economics and Government, founded in 1924.

The Board of Trustees is responsible for the general administration of the Institution, while the immediate direction of the policies, program, and staff is vested in the President, assisted by an advisory committee of the officers and staff. The by-laws of the Institution state: "It is the function of the Trustees to make possible the conduct of scientific research, and publication, under the most favorable conditions, and to safeguard the independence of the research staff in the pursuit of their studies and in the publication of the results of such studies. It is not a part of their function to determine, control, or influence the conduct of particular investigations or the conclusions reached."

The President bears final responsibility for the decision to publish a manuscript as a Brookings book. In reaching his judgment on the competence, accuracy, and objectivity of each study, the President is advised by the director of the appropriate research program and weighs the views of a panel of expert outside readers who report to him in confidence on the quality of the work. Publication of a work signifies that it is deemed a competent treatment worthy of public consideration but does not imply endorsement of conclusions or recommendations.

The Institution maintains its position of neutrality on issues of public policy in order to safeguard the intellectual freedom of the staff. Hence interpretations or conclusions in Brookings publications should be understood to be solely those of the authors and should not be attributed to the Institution, to its trustees, officers, or other staff members, or to the organizations that support its research.

Foreword

Americans spend billions of dollars a year on medical care, much of it in attempts to cure diseases that are already far advanced. Heart disease and cancer—conditions that usually do not appear until late in life—have become the major killers. They remain largely unconquered despite important advances in therapy and in our understanding of their causes. Part of that understanding is the growing realization that these illnesses of later life are often caused by habits formed years earlier. Smoking is firmly established as a cause of lung disease, including cancer; more recent evidence shows it to be a cause of heart disease as well. Several studies suggest that diet and exercise are linked to both heart disease and cancer. As good cures continue to elude us, attention has turned to the possibility that prevention may be the most effective tool for good health during middle and old age.

This volume summarizes the proceedings of a workshop held at the Brookings Institution on May 8 and 9, 1986, to assess the potential of prevention for improving the health of older people. The participants—twenty-seven experts in medicine, epidemiology, and methods of evaluation—were asked to decide whether the evidence about the effects of prevention on health in six areas was good enough to warrant more careful, sophisticated attempts to evaluate the cost-effectiveness of change. The six areas are drug therapy for high blood pressure, smoking, exercise, dietary calcium, alcohol use, and obesity. In the course of a wide-ranging, probing discussion, the participants decided that smoking, hypertension, and perhaps exercise were ready for further evaluation, while the possibilities for good evaluations in the other areas were limited.

Louise B. Russell, a senior fellow in the Economic Studies program at Brookings, organized the workshop and authored this summary. Financing was provided by a grant from the Office for Income Security Policy in the Office of the Assistant Secretary for Planning and Evaluation, Department of Health and Human Services. The workshop was put together after consultations with many people. Particular thanks are owed to Michele Adler, Donald Berwick, Jeffery A. Cutler, Gordon DeFriese, Suzanne Fletcher, Hellen Gelband, James Harrell, Philip Lee, Bill Lohr, Kathleen Lohr, Kenneth E. Powell, Richard S. Rivlin, Jane E. Sisk, Albert J. Stunkard, Richard Suzman, Gregg Thomas, Ernestine Vanderveen, and Milton C. Weinstein. Dawn Emery handled the logistics of the workshop.

The manuscript was reviewed by the workshop participants. Thomas Turner kindly consented to review part of the manuscript as well. Theresa B. Walker edited the manuscript, and Carrie L. Manning and Almaz S. Zelleke checked the manuscript for factual accuracy. Alice Fins prepared the index.

The views expressed in this volume are those of the workshop participants and should not be ascribed to the trustees, officers, or other staff members of the Brookings Institution, to the Office for Income Security Policy, or to any of those who were consulted about the workshop.

April 1987
Washington, D.C.

BRUCE K. MAC LAURY
President

Contents

chapter one **Introduction**

Poor health is an important element in older people's decision to retire. It can reduce their capacity for work even before retirement, and thus their earnings, and prevent them from working part time to supplement their pensions after retirement. The medical expenses and premature disability that may result from a severe illness can have a devastating impact on the financial well-being of an older individual. While disabling conditions can strike at any time in life, they are particularly likely to strike older people.

Prevention offers a promising avenue for improving the health of people in middle and old age. A growing body of evidence indicates that some of the major causes of illness and disability can be prevented either through specific interventions, such as drugs to control high blood pressure, or through general changes in diet, exercise, smoking, and other personal habits. The adoption of these changes by individuals may have significant effects on their ability to cope with growing older, the number of elderly people in poverty, and the financial demands on government programs.

The Workshop

On May 8 and 9, 1986, the Brookings Institution held a workshop to consider the state of information on the cost-effectiveness of prevention as a way to improve older people's capacity to work. The workshop was the first phase of a plan to evaluate major preventive strategies to determine which are likely to have the greatest effects on health and capacity to

This introduction draws on the closing remarks made at the workshop by *Alice M. Rivlin* and *Henry Blackburn.* In his remarks *Blackburn* briefly reviewed each session, which helped to shape the organization of chapters 2 through 8.

work, relative to their costs. Six areas were examined: drug therapy for hypertension, smoking, exercise, dietary calcium, alcohol use, and obesity. All six have important consequences for the health of the nation.

To understand these consequences better it is necessary to consider more carefully how preventive efforts might affect people's health and capacity to work as they age. For example, in the Social Security Amendments of 1983 Congress agreed to raise the age at which retirees could receive full benefits under social security. Starting in the year 2000, that age will increase gradually from the current 65 years until it reaches 67 years in 2022. For current retirees such a change could represent considerable hardship since many of them are already in poor health at age 65. But with life expectancies increasing and health improving, it may cause substantially fewer problems for retirees of the year 2000 and beyond. The health of future retirees will be created in part by the preventive practices adopted today.

Two kinds of studies are potentially helpful: those that project the health improvements from prevention and describe their consequences for the capacity to work, without specifying how to achieve them; and those that specify a particular way to achieve the improvements, such as a change in the minimum drinking age, and estimate the costs of the intervention as well as its effects on the capacity to work. The first is a partial, the second a complete, cost-effectiveness analysis. Both types of studies require much the same kinds of information about health and much the same kinds of methods for analyzing the implications of change.

Evidence about health is the starting point for either kind of analysis. The consequences of a disease or habit must be serious, and intervention must be effective in reducing those consequences, before it is worthwhile to evaluate the cost-effectiveness of change. For these reasons the workshop focused on evaluating information about the health effects of change in each of the six areas. It would be worthwhile to proceed with an analysis only if that information is reasonably complete and indicates that change would be effective.

A second step is required when the focus is on capacity to work. Most evidence about the health effects of prevention is expressed in deaths and cases of disease avoided—heart disease, cancer, diabetes, osteoporosis, and the like. What a disease means for everyday life, however, depends on the degree of disability that accompanies it—whether it causes pain, fatigue, difficulty in walking, and the like. The disease needs to be described in terms of its effects on ability to function, particularly in ways important for holding a job, before the implications of prevention can be made clear. The workshop also addressed methods for translating the usual kinds of evidence about health into measures of the capacity to work.

The same data and methods lend themselves to the analysis of important issues other than capacity to work. Better health improves the well-being of older people and their overall ability to function, to live independently, and to care for themselves. For all these subjects, evidence on the health effects of change is essential. The methods for translating changes in the incidence of particular diseases into changes in overall health and ability to function are as necessary for these issues as for income security issues. Thus the findings of the workshop apply to a wide range of policy issues, not just those that were the primary reason for holding it.

The workshop was not undertaken with the expectation that, when analyses are ultimately done, they will show that prevention saves money. Most evaluations to date have examined medical expenditures and have shown that prevention adds to those expenditures, at the same time, of course, that it adds to health.[1] If future analyses show that prevention will reduce expenditures, overall or in some areas, well and good. But savings are not a prerequisite for taking prevention seriously. Better health is worth paying for. It allows people to enjoy life, to help others, and to live independently, as well as to contribute to their own support. These outcomes are valuable whether or not they are accompanied by savings.

While cost-effectiveness analysis can be, and has been, used to estimate whether proposed programs will save money, its uses go well beyond that question. Simply put, cost-effectiveness analysis is a set of methods for determining the effects of a proposed change and the costs necessary to achieve those effects. The change is cost-effective whenever the effects are considered worth the costs, not only when they are free because the savings outweigh the costs. Thus cost-effectiveness can help the nation choose those investments that bring the most health for the required expenditure.

---

1. See Russell 1986 in the bibliography under "Guidelines for Cost-Effectiveness Evaluations."

Plan of the Book

A cost-effectiveness evaluation compares the costs of prevention with its health effects. *Costs* are usually fairly readily measured in dollars and include the costs of the intervention and the costs of treating any side effects caused by the intervention. Health effects, which were the focus of the workshop, measure the improvements in health brought about by the intervention (for example, the improvements brought about by using seat belts). *Health effects* are the sum of the years of life added by the intervention; and the improvements in health during years that would have been lived anyway; minus any deterioration in health because of side effects of the intervention.

Three kinds of information are required to do a complete cost-effectiveness evaluation of prevention as a way to improve work capacity: information on the health effects of the condition to be changed; information about the effectiveness, side effects, and costs of intervening to change the condition; and methods to translate estimates of disease into estimates of capacity to work and ability to function.

All three elements were covered by the workshop. The sessions followed a traditional format—a background paper was presented and then discussed. The author of the paper reviewed methods or information essential to the modeling of health effects, and the discussants then considered how well the methods or information met the needs of a cost-effectiveness analysis. Particularly in the sessions on smoking, exercise, dietary calcium, alcohol use, and obesity, however, the discussants had an untraditional role to play. Their job was to engage the author of the paper and each other in a conversation about the evidence, as if they were planning to undertake a cost-effectiveness analysis together, in order to decide whether an analysis was feasible.

This book is a summary of the workshop proceedings. The important outcome of the workshop was the conclusions that emerged from the interchange among the participants rather than the individual presentations. The summary of each session is therefore not a strictly chronological record. Instead it organizes and emphasizes the evidence to reflect the final conclusions.

Chapter 2 describes the modeling of health effects for an evaluation that has already been done, the classic study of drug therapy for hypertension (high blood pressure) by Milton C. Weinstein and William B. Stason. Although the information in an area may be very good, it is never perfect, and this example shows how information from different sources and of differing quality can be combined to produce an analysis that has stood the test of time well. The study gives a realistic sense for the amount of information that is necessary for a cost-effectiveness analysis. Further, it illustrates, in the context of a specific example, how to piece together data from various sources. With this example in mind, it was easier for the workshop participants, and should be easier for the reader of the book, to decide whether the information about other areas of prevention is capable of supporting cost-effectiveness analyses.

Anyone who wanted to extend the analysis of hypertension to show its implications for capacity to work would need some methods for translating changes in the incidence of heart disease and stroke into improvements in ability to function. Chapter 3 discusses these methods. The first set of methods described in the chapter relates specific diseases to overall patterns of function that are clearly relevant to individuals' ability to work. The second set of methods addresses the problem of comparing and valuing different patterns of function; the methods have been applied to general health outcomes but could be used to value capacity to work.

Chapters 2 and 3 give important background for assessing the adequacy of the information about the five remaining areas: smoking, exercise, dietary calcium, alcohol use, and obesity. Chapters 4 through 8 review these areas, using two sets of questions to guide each review. The first set of questions asks:

—What are the health effects of the condition, for example, smoking, and how severe are they? How solid is the evidence? What are the effects on other people, for example, from passive smoking or alcohol-related traffic accidents?

—Do the health effects have the potential to affect capacity to work in important ways, either because of their nature or because of the groups involved, or both?

The second set of questions addresses possible interventions to change the conditions:

—Do effective ways to intervene exist? How effective are they? Are some methods more appropriate for improving work capacity?

—What are the side effects of intervention, particularly any adverse health effects?

—How much is known about the costs of intervention? Although the participants were not asked to spend much time on this subject, they did mention some of the costs that should be considered and something of what is known about those costs.

Comparisons are the essence of cost-effectiveness analyses. Analyses compare the costs and effects of alternative interventions. To help in making comparisons, cost-effectiveness evaluations of different interventions should be based as much as possible on the same principles and basic assumptions. The appendix recommends guidelines for cost-effectiveness evaluations.

Conclusions

The workshop reaffirmed the great potential of prevention for lengthening life and improving health. For smoking, the evidence of destructive effects on health, and of the benefits of quitting or never starting, is overwhelmingly convincing. In other areas, the scientific evidence is growing rapidly. Some benefits are well established, such as the effects of exercise on heart disease. Others, such as the effects of exercise on bone strength, are only suggested by the studies now available.

The workshop also showed that the framework for evaluating prevention is reasonably complete. Cost-effectiveness has been successfully applied to such areas as drug therapy for hypertension. Methods exist for translating outcomes expressed in terms of disease into outcomes expressed in terms of ability to function. Other methods allow the outcomes to be valued and compared. Although there is room for improvement and refinement of these methods, the basic building blocks are available. Cost-effectiveness analysis, together with the methods for projecting health effects and translating them into information about capacity to work, provides a coherent framework for organizing the available information and working out its implications.

The reviews in part 2 suggest that cost-effectiveness evaluations could usefully be done of changes in smoking, exercise, and obesity, and their effects on capacity to work. A comprehensive analysis of smoking may be possible. For exercise and obesity, the analyses may have to focus on particular conditions or subgroups. The study of hypertension, already done, could be updated and extended to examine the issue of capacity to work.

For the use of alcohol and for dietary calcium, cost-effectiveness analyses may not be justified at this time, although not everyone at the workshop would agree. For alcohol use, the participants disagreed over the adequacy and interpretation of the data, and thus over their recommendations about the area's readiness for evaluation. For dietary calcium, considerable uncertainty still exists about how and when calcium strengthens the bone structure, thus preventing fractures in old age. Further, this area illustrates, perhaps more pointedly than the others, the growing realization that each change affects many diseases, and each disease has many causes. Analysts need to begin to consider how to integrate the information based on single causes and diseases into a more comprehensive picture of prevention and health. A cost-effectiveness evaluation that attempted this integration would be a major contribution.

In none of these areas is the information complete, nor will it ever be. Cost-effectiveness can help here as well by showing which gaps are most important. When there is considerable doubt about some item thought to be important, the analysis can be done for all the likely values. For example, if the side effects of an intervention are largely unknown, the analysis can be done once assuming that they are negligible and again assuming that they are more important. If the results are very different for the two assumptions, additional information about side effects is important. If not, the additional information may not be worth the effort to collect.

It is important not to set the standards for evaluations unrealistically high. It will always be necessary to make assumptions in order to analyze alternative policies. The information will always be weak in some respects. At the same time, many decisions are made on the basis of information much less complete than that presented at the workshop. The information already available for many areas of prevention is good enough to warrant careful and complete analyses that will reveal to individuals and policymakers the implications of the choices open to them, as well as the probable effects of choices already made.

part one   **Modeling Health Effects and Work Capacity**

Marilyn Bergner
Jeffrey A. Cutler
Robert M. Kaplan
Stephen MacMahon
Kenneth G. Manton
Donald L. Patrick
Daniel D. Savage
Milton C. Weinstein

chapter two   **How to Model Health Effects:**
The Case of Hypertension

In 1976, Milton C. Weinstein and William B. Stason
published *Hypertension: A Policy Perspective,* a cost-effectiveness analysis of screening and drug therapy for hypertension.[1] At that time the
evidence showing that drugs to lower blood pressure could save lives and
prevent disease was still fairly new. The Veterans' Administration trials,
which demonstrated the benefits of drugs for men with moderate or severe
hypertension, had been published in 1967 and 1970. The results of those
trials were, however, so impressive that a national initiative had been
undertaken to encourage people to seek treatment. In the hope that drugs
would also be beneficial for mild hypertension, a major trial—the U.S.
Hypertension Detection and Follow-up Program, which enrolled more
than 10,000 people—was under way, although results were not yet available.[2]

Major decisions were being made about the medical care of millions of
people, and substantial amounts of resources were being committed on the
basis of those decisions. Using the information available, Weinstein and
Stason carried out their analysis to determine what was being gained and at
what cost. They evaluated the cost-effectiveness of screening and treatment for men and women at different ages and with different degrees of
hypertension, including mild hypertension. Their results showed that, in
1975, drug therapy averaged $4,850 per year of life gained for those with
moderate or severe hypertension; screening brought the cost to $7,000 per
year. The cost varied considerably by age and sex and by whether the

---

Milton C. Weinstein wrote and presented the background paper. *Stephen MacMahon,
Jeffrey A. Cutler,* and *Daniel D. Savage* were the discussants.
    1. Weinstein and Stason 1976; also 1978.
    2. Hypertension Detection and Follow-up Program Cooperative Group 1979.

patient took the drugs faithfully or not. The costs were higher for people with mild hypertension.[3]

At the workshop Weinstein described how he and Stason modeled health effects for the analysis. Although a great deal of information had accumulated about hypertension, they had to make several assumptions and piece together evidence from various sources, ranging from large, well-designed studies to expert opinion. Their experience offers a useful guide to other analysts considering cost-effectiveness analyses.

The Model of Health Effects

Weinstein and Stason took the social perspective for their analysis and counted all costs, no matter who paid them, and all health effects, no matter who experienced them. The cost per year of life gained was calculated on the basis of the following formula:

$$\text{cost per year} = \frac{\text{net costs}}{\text{net health effects}}$$

Net costs are the total of the costs of treatment; minus savings in medical costs because heart attacks and strokes are prevented; plus the costs of treating side effects of the drugs; plus ordinary medical costs in years of life added by the treatment.[4] Net health effects are the sum of three elements: years of life added by drug therapy; plus improvements in health because of therapy (valued in an equivalent number of years of life); minus the side effects of the drugs (also valued in an equivalent number of years of life).

3. Blood pressure is measured at two points during the heart's cycle of contraction and relaxation and hypertension can be, and is, defined in terms of the higher (systolic) pressure, the lower (diastolic) pressure, or a combination of the two. The definition most commonly used depends on the diastolic pressure and divides the range into normal (less than 90), mild hypertension (90–104), moderate hypertension (105–114), and severe hypertension (115 or higher). A recent report from an ad hoc committee of the World Health Organization and the International Society of Hypertension modified these definitions to exclude from mild hypertension patients with signs of damage to the heart or other organs as a consequence of high blood pressure (World Health Organization 1986).

4. The last item is appropriate if the analysis is concerned with whether the intervention raises or lowers total medical expenditures. If, instead, it is concerned simply with whether the intervention is a good use of resources, either all indirect costs should be included, or none should be (medical expenditures in years of life added by the intervention are an indirect cost). See the Appendix.

Information about the health effects of hypertension and the effectiveness of drugs in treating it is clearly essential for estimating net health effects. The same information was also necessary to estimate costs. For example, savings in medical costs can only be calculated with the aid of data on the number of heart attacks and strokes prevented by drug therapy. Similarly, the costs of treating side effects required knowledge of the kinds of side effects associated with the drugs.

Hypertension is widespread. As much as 20 percent of the adult population suffers from it in some degree. The primary consequences of hypertension are stroke and heart attack, which usually come late in life, often when they influence retirement decisions and limit people's ability to work after retirement. Most hypertension is mild; about one-third of hypertensive individuals suffer from moderate or severe hypertension.

The first task in the modeling effort was to quantify the relationship between blood pressure and its two primary health effects, strokes and heart attacks. The data for this purpose came from the Framingham study, which has tracked cardiovascular disease in much of the population of Framingham, Massachusetts, for more than two decades.[5] The study provided excellent evidence for that relationship because of the large number of people followed and because those selected for the study were free of cardiovascular disease at the outset. The investigators at Framingham had found that the data fit a logistic curve, one in which the risk of death or illness increases at an increasing rate as blood pressure rises. Put another way, a ten-point increase in blood pressure is associated with a larger rise in the death rate for someone whose initial pressure is 110 than for someone whose initial pressure is 95. For their analysis, Weinstein and Stason fitted separate curves of the same type for each age and sex group.

The next step was to model the effectiveness of intervention. The Veterans' Administration trials had only shown drugs to be effective for moderate and severe hypertension. Weinstein and Stason calculated that the VA trials had been too small to produce statistically significant effects for mild hypertension, even if such effects existed. They decided to assume for their analysis that mild hypertensives would benefit from drugs.

They then had to develop some assumptions about the size of the benefit. They figured the most optimistic possibility was that lowering blood pressure with drugs made someone just as healthy as a person who

5. This study has produced many publications. For a recent summary of many of the findings, see Dawber 1980.

had that blood pressure naturally; they called this the assumption of full
benefit. It was the most optimistic assumption, but not, they thought, the
most likely. It seemed more likely that the benefit was some fraction of
full benefit and that the fraction depended on the length of time the drugs
were taken and the age at which they were started, with the benefit greater
for those who started young, before their hypertension had time to cause
damage.

The statistical evidence was not sufficient to permit calculation of this
"fraction of benefit" for different ages and different lengths of treatment,
so Weinstein and Stason asked several experts for their opinions. The
experts helped them create a table of values showing how close to full
benefit each age/treatment group could reasonably hope to come. The
table of values, labeled the assumption of "age-varying partial benefit"
was used for most of the analysis. Additional calculations were made for
the case of full benefit.

Weinstein and Stason now had most of the elements needed to estimate
the additional years of life and the reduced rates of nonfatal disease that
drugs could produce. They knew about how many people suffered from
the various degrees of hypertension and what their risks of disease and
death were compared with those of normal people. They had tables of
values allowing them to estimate how far individuals' blood pressure could
be reduced and how close that reduction would bring them to the death and
disease rates of normal people (the fraction of benefit).

To complete the calculation of the first health effect and most of the
calculation of the second, they needed one more item—the rates of death,
stroke, and heart attack in the population. The rates observed in the
Framingham population were not appropriate because that population was
healthier than average. Instead, Weinstein and Stason applied the relationship estimated from the Framingham data to national death and disease
rates.

To complete the second and third items, they also needed some way to
value improvements or side effects in the same units as additions to years
of life. For this they used the method of the quality-adjusted life-year,
sometimes called the well-year or the year of healthy life, which is detailed in chapter 3. This method assumes that people have some idea of
how many days of life with poor health they would be willing to give up in
order to have good health. For example, someone with emphysema might
be willing to give up a month of life for every year with that condition in
order to have good health instead. If the year of good health is given the

value 1.0, the year with emphysema would thus be worth .917 of a year to that person. Any intervention that eliminated the emphysema would receive credit for .083 of a year of life for every year of emphysema prevented. Using assumptions like these, Weinstein and Stason valued the improvements in health and the adverse effects of drugs in terms of years of life gained or lost. This method allowed them to express all the health effects in years of healthy life and to sum them.

The assumption made for side effects turned out to be especially important. Weinstein and Stason knew that side effects were common, although there were no data showing how common. They also knew side effects were generally mild or of short duration. They decided to assume that a year on drugs was worth .99 of a healthy year because of the side effects; thus the average person would be willing to give up .01 of a year, or just under four days, to avoid them. They tested the alternative assumptions that a year on drugs was equal to a year of good health, and that it was worth only .98 of a healthy year. The calculations showed that when side effects reduced the value of a year by eight days, the cost of a healthy year increased considerably because the net gains from treatment were smaller.

The modeling of health effects included other features of the relationships between hypertension, disease, and drug therapy. For example, the authors built into the model the well-established fact that blood pressure rises as people grow older and the assumption that treatment moderates the rise.[6]

When the model was complete, Weinstein and Stason tested their estimates of the extra years to be gained by people of different ages and initial blood pressures against the estimates of other analysts. When they were satisfied that their calculations were reasonable they proceeded with the cost estimation and the final calculations of cost per year of life gained.

As noted earlier, their results showed that the cost of treatment in 1975 came to $4,850 per year of life gained for people with moderate or severe hypertension, $7,000 if the cost of screening to identify these individuals is included. The results varied considerably with the patient's age, sex, and initial blood pressure, and also with whether the patient took the medication exactly as prescribed or omitted it some of the time. The cost per year of life was lower for those with higher initial pressures, meaning that it was more cost-effective to treat them. It was lower for older than for

6. A more detailed discussion of the modeling is given in chap. 2 of Weinstein and Stason 1976.

younger women, but the reverse was true for men—the cost was lower for young men. When patients did not take the drug as prescribed and so did not achieve full benefit, the cost per year of life gained rose into the $15,000 to $20,000 range.

Developments since Completion of the Model

Since the publication of Weinstein and Stason's study, the results from several major clinical trials of drug therapy for mild hypertension have become public. Besides the Hypertension Detection and Follow-up Program in the United States, there are the Australian trial, which followed about 3,500 men and women, the British Medical Research Council Trial, which followed 17,000 people, and other, smaller studies.[7]

Collectively, the trials supported Weinstein and Stason's assumption that drugs benefit people with mild hypertension. Most of the major trials showed that mild hypertensives treated with drugs had lower death rates than those who did not receive drugs.

The implications of the trials for the maximum benefit that can be achieved are not agreed on, but the possibilities are interesting and not entirely in accord with the assumption of age-varying partial benefit. Weinstein and Stason have calculated that the fraction of benefit experienced in these trials may be greater than 1.0, that is, that someone whose hypertension is controlled with drugs may be better off than someone with a natural blood pressure of the same level.

Jeffrey A. Cutler and Stephen MacMahon have calculated the fraction of benefit separately for stroke and heart disease. Their results show that the fraction of benefit for stroke is at least 1.0, that is, that full benefit is achieved, and that it is achieved within six years of beginning drugs, so that the assumption that benefit varies with length of treatment is not valid after six years. For heart disease, they think the fraction of benefit is in the range of 0.4 to 0.6—only about half the full benefit—and the possibility that there is no benefit at all cannot yet be ruled out. Further, it is not clear whether the benefit increases with the length of treatment; the nature of heart disease and some of the physiological side effects of antihypertensive drugs suggest that it may not.

In a related finding, the trials also suggest that treatment may not be

7. Hypertension Detection and Follow-up Program Cooperative Group 1979; Management Committee 1980; and Medical Research Council Working Party 1985.

more effective when started at younger ages. While epidemiological data, such as that from Framingham, suggest that the health gains should be greater for younger men, the data from the trials do not show the expected differences. Why this should be so is not clear, but it may be because relative rates of stroke and heart disease differ among age groups or because older people are more conscientious about taking medication. Then again, it may simply result from the fact that, large as they were, the trials were not large enough to produce definitive results for subgroups.

Much more is known about the prevalence and nature of side effects. Recent data suggest that as many as 20 percent of those taking antihypertensive drugs suffer them.[8] The information about subjective side effects, those that people actually experience, needs to be translated into the terms used by Weinstein and Stason before it will be possible to see how the information might alter the results. Metabolic side effects, those that show up primarily or only in laboratory tests, may have important implications for the long-term effects of drugs on death and disease, but these implications are not yet known.

Daniel D. Savage indicated that a new test—echocardiography—is producing a more complete picture of hypertension.[9] Echocardiograms are a noninvasive method for estimating the weight of the left ventricle, the main pumping chamber of the heart. Recent studies suggest that abnormal increases in this weight (left ventricular hypertrophy) identify people at particular risk from hypertension[10] and those vulnerable to the side effects of certain antihypertensive medications.[11] Some research indicates that weight loss may be important for overweight hypertensives with left ventricular hypertrophy; in some of these people, weight loss may eliminate the need for drugs.[12] As the information in this area accumulates, it may be possible to estimate a new logistic curve relating blood pressure to disease and death that identifies risks and appropriate therapy more precisely.

Several items of cost have changed since Weinstein and Stason did their analysis and might change the results. It is less common now to search for

8. Medical Research Council Working Party 1981.
9. Savage, Abbott, Padget, and others 1983; and Savage, Drayer, Henry, and others 1979.
10. Savage, Garrison, Castelli, and others 1985; and Casale, Devereux, Milner, and others 1986.
11. Topol, Traill, and Fortuin 1986; and Savage, Castelli, Abbott, and others 1983.
12. MacMahon, Wilcken, and Macdonald 1986; and Joint National Committee on Detection, Evaluation, and Treatment of High Blood Pressure 1984.

a specific cause for hypertension during the patient's diagnostic workup, perhaps as a result of Weinstein and Stason's finding that it cost a lot but produced little benefit. New antihypertensive drugs are more expensive than those commonly used when they did their research. The treatment of heart attack has changed, with shorter hospital stays but more intensive care.

One of the most interesting new possibilities for analysis is raised by trials suggesting that it may not be necessary to take drugs continuously throughout life to control high blood pressure. At least some people may be able to take drugs intermittently, with drug-taking periods followed by "drug holidays." Intermittent drug schedules could reduce both the cost and side effects of drug treatment without sacrificing the health benefits.

The discussion confirmed that, overall, the analysis has stood the test of time well. It accurately reflected the medical and epidemiological evidence of the time—the evidence on which medical decisions were being made—and even included some assumptions about items for which no statistical evidence was then available that were later proved correct. In other cases, the recent trials point to some of the alternatives that were analyzed as more likely than others, or they raise questions about the assumptions (for example, the assumption that benefit increases with the length of treatment). And new conditions and new possibilities suggest it may soon be possible to evaluate alternatives not considered in 1975. One change that would clearly produce different results if an analysis were done today is the substantial decline in deaths from heart disease during the last decade. Nonetheless, the overall impression of most analysts is that the updated model of health effects would not be very different from the model put together in 1975.

To help analysts considering other preventive interventions, Weinstein outlined what he thinks is the minimum information needed to model health effects. He suggested that randomized controlled trials are rarely large enough to support quantitative estimates for the model; instead they are often best used for their qualitative conclusions, with the quantitative estimates drawn from large epidemiological data sets like the Framingham study. With that point in mind, he suggested two essential elements for a cost-effectiveness study. First, at least one good study must show the proportional reduction in death or disease for a given change in the precursor condition (for example, high blood pressure or smoking). Second, epidemiological data on the rates of disease and death in the population must be available. For hypertension, the Framingham study provided the first. The second was derived from national vital statistics.

chapter three

How to Translate Health Effects into Work Capacity

Medical studies measure health effects in terms of death and types of disease—heart disease, stroke, cancer, arthritis, and the like. For evaluations concerned primarily with the capacity to work, these effects need to be translated into terms that indicate how much the disease affects individuals' ability to work. If lives are saved, are people capable of working during the added years? If health is improved, does the improvement bring with it a greater capacity for work? A focus on capacity to work means that only some of the benefits of longer life and better health are of direct interest for the evaluation.

The translation requires two steps. Changes in disease must first be linked to changes in capacity to work. The changes in capacity to work must then be valued in some common unit that allows different kinds of change to be compared. At the workshop Kenneth G. Manton discussed methods for linking disease to capacity to work. He also reviewed methods for relating risk factors such as hypertension, smoking, or obesity to disease, an essential task for any cost-effectiveness study of health, whatever its ultimate focus. Robert M. Kaplan described methods for valuing health effects, which could be adapted to value different levels or types of work capacity.

Whether an individual works depends not only on health or ability to work but also on whether opportunities for work are available and on willingness to work. The three cannot always be distinguished clearly—willingness can affect ability, ability can affect opportunities, and so on. But changes in rates of disease have the most to do with ability or capacity

---

Kenneth G. Manton wrote and presented the paper on linking disease to the capacity to work. *Robert M. Kaplan* wrote and presented the paper about valuing different types of capacity to work; John P. Anderson was the coauthor. *Marilyn Bergner* and *Donald L. Patrick* discussed the papers.

to work, and the workshop focused on this aspect of work. Work was defined broadly to include producing products or services for others, whether or not the worker was paid. Thus the aim is to show how and when changes in health affect people's ability to produce goods and services for others—to perform work useful for society—either as volunteers or as paid members of the labor force.[1]

Linking Disease to Capacity to Work

Manton began by reviewing some general methods for modeling health effects in traditional terms. To do this the analyst needs to describe the relationship of the risk factor to disease and death at any point in time and the change in the risk factor, or factors, over time as the individual ages. With these two elements, it is then possible to project when a condition, such as high blood pressure, will result in death or disease. Milton C. Weinstein described the methods he and William B. Stason used to accomplish this modeling for their study of hypertension. The methods proposed by Manton serve the same purpose but differ in detail and are suitable for a variety of risk factors.

Modeling Health Effects in Traditional Terms

The first element essential to the traditional model of health effects is the relationship between the risk factors and the adverse effect, disease or death.[2] Calling this the "hazard function," Manton proposed a form in which each disease is a function of the same risk factors. This form recognizes that diseases are not independent. A given risk factor may influence several diseases, and an individual who does not develop one disease may develop another associated with the same risk factor.

The general function specifies a quadratic term for each risk factor, reflecting a relationship between risk factor and disease that has been found in many cases—that is, both unusually high and unusually low values of the risk factor are associated with higher rates of disease. The function can also include interactions among risk factors to reflect situa-

1. Even when an improvement in health is not enough to make the individual capable of working, it may—if the individual can take over more of his or her own care—free someone else to do other work.
2. See Woodbury and Manton 1977; and Manton 1986.

tions in which the adverse effects of the two together are worse than the sum of their separate effects.

Manton recommended that the hazard function also incorporate the general rise in rates of disease and death with age. This can be done in at least two ways. Age can be included as a separate variable in the function, or the entire function can be multiplied by a term that reflects an appropriate change with age. The Gompertz function is one such term and, in his work, Manton has found that it produces more realistic patterns of change with age than the first alternative.[3]

The second element of the traditional model is a description of the changes in risk factors as individuals age. Manton proposed a simple equation relating each risk factor to its own past value and a change term dependent on age. The error term in the equation means that both the mean and the variance of the risk factor can be projected.

Manton applied these methods to data from the Framingham study. He then used the estimated equations to calculate the increased life expectancy that might result from programs to control cholesterol, blood sugar, cigarette smoking, hypertension, and vital capacity. Three types of programs were tested in the analysis—programs to reduce the rise in the risk factor with age; programs to reduce the variance in the risk factor, that is, to reduce the values of those individuals at the extremes; and programs to reduce both the rise and the extreme values.

The general conclusion that came out of these experiments was an interesting one with particular significance for the capacity to work. Programs to reduce extreme values of the risk factors, without attempting to change the rise with age, increased the life expectancy of younger people—those in their 30s, 40s, and 50s—somewhat more than that of older people, while controlling the rise with age had about the same effect for all age groups. Donald L. Patrick pointed out that individuals with extreme values tend to be the poor and minority groups, so that a program aimed at reducing the extremes would be directed at a very different population from one that tried to hold down the rise with age.

Moving from Disease to Work Capacity

Manton tackled the problem of describing the effects of disease on capacity to work in two steps. He first analyzed data on disabilities to

3. For more about the Gompertz function, see Spiegelman 1969.

identify general patterns of disability with clear implications for capacity to work. Then he linked those general patterns to the specific diseases associated with them.

To identify patterns of disability he turned to data from the 1982 National Long-Term Care Survey. This survey included information about 6,400 people aged 65 or older who were chronically disabled but not in institutions; a disability was defined as chronic if it had existed for at least ninety days at the time of the survey. Nationally, about 5 million of the 26 million to 27 million people over 65 years of age in 1982 were in this category—chronically disabled but not in institutions. Manton argued that this group is the logical target for preventive programs aimed at improving capacity to work. It omits those in institutions and those who have chronic disease, such as heart disease, but no significant chronic disability yet associated with it.

The survey provided extensive information on the limitations of these people. The questionnaire asked each individual about his or her ability to perform certain "activities of daily living (ADLs)," a standard series of activities widely used to assess disability. The basic ADLs check whether the individual is confined to bed or a wheelchair and whether he or she needs help with eating, dressing, bathing, using the toilet, and getting around inside the house. A second set—the "instrumental activities of daily living"—probes the limitations of less severely disabled people, asking whether they need help with household tasks such as laundry and grocery shopping, with managing money, taking medicine, and making telephone calls. A third set of questions probes the difficulty the individual has with specific physical activities—climbing stairs, combing hair, holding a ten-pound package, and the like.

Manton discovered that the twenty-seven specific limitations tended to cluster in groups. Using a type of factor analysis, he identified five major patterns of disability.[4] The first was a relatively healthy group with few limitations and considerable ability to perform heavy work. The second group had significant problems with moving around, especially outside. The third had a wider range of physical difficulties, but, like the second, showed no signs of cognitive impairment. The fourth group had few physical limitations but serious cognitive limitations—they were unable to travel, manage money, make phone calls, or do housework without help.

4. Woodbury and Manton 1982.

The fifth and final group was a very seriously disabled group with limitations in virtually every category.

The first three groups, and certainly the first, should be capable of performing some kinds of work. For the second and third groups, the work would need to be tailored to their physical limitations. The fourth and fifth groups would not be capable of working.

The distribution of 67-year-olds in the survey gives a sense for the relative importance of the five groups. Sixty-seven is a particularly interesting age to examine because after the year 2000 it will be phased in as the official retirement age, the age at which individuals are eligible for full social security benefits. In 1982, 31 percent of this noninstitutionalized, disabled population were relatively healthy and thus fell in the first group. Twenty-one percent fell in the second group, with limited mobility; 19 percent in the more physically limited third group; 11 percent in the group with serious cognitive limitations; and 17 percent in the very disabled group.

With the five groups identified, Manton turned to the problem of linking these patterns of disability to the diseases that cause them. For this he used the coefficients produced by the factor analysis. These coefficients showed the strength of the relationships between each of the limitations reported by an individual and the five major disability groups. Manton used regression analysis to estimate the relationships between these coefficients and twelve types of disease, including heart attack, cancer, stroke, and rheumatism. In the regressions each disease was represented by a binary variable indicating that it was or was not present. The binaries were multiplied by the age of the individual so that the analysis produced a set of relationships unique to each year of age.

Once these regressions were estimated, it was possible to move back and forth between diseases and the major disability groups to determine how changes in the prevalence of a particular disease would change the number of people in each group. Manton illustrated the possibilities with some calculations relating the two for 67-year-olds. The results suggested that if all twelve diseases were eliminated, the healthy group would increase from 31 percent of the total to 48 percent. The gains came from reductions in groups three and five; the other two groups were basically unaffected.

The results also suggested that reducing hip fractures, stroke, and senility would have the greatest impact on disability, although other diseases and conditions were also important. Two of those conditions are closely related to areas of prevention considered at the workshop. Hip fractures are caused by osteoporosis, which dietary calcium may prevent. Strokes are strongly related to hypertension, which can be controlled by drugs. The results should not, however, be taken as definitive since they apply only to 67-year-olds, and the same patterns may not show up at older ages.

It is important to keep in mind that the analysis excludes older people in nursing homes and other institutions. Some of these people are there because of disabilities that might be delayed or eliminated by prevention. In fact, the differences between these people and some of the most severely disabled in the community is less their disabilities than the availability of friends, relatives, and money to support them at home.

The analysis also excludes the possibility that eliminating certain diseases might eliminate all disabilities for some people, putting them in the population of those elderly without chronic disabilities. A complete analysis will need to consider how prevention might move people from the institutionalized population to the disabled population in the community, and from the disabled population in the community to the population without chronic disabilities. The methods outlined by Manton could be extended to handle these shifts among groups.

Valuing Different Types of Capacity to Work

Suppose that one preventive intervention reduces the number of people in the second disability group and moves them into the first, while another intervention reduces the numbers of people in groups four and five, moving them into groups two and three. Faced with these results, how would the administrator of a program decide which intervention was the better investment? If the administrator did it intuitively, he or she would value the results of the two programs on some intuitive common scale and, weighing the costs and other considerations as well, choose the one he or she preferred, much the way people decide which car to buy or which medical advice to follow.

For public policy decisions, it is helpful to develop an explicit process for valuing the outcomes of different interventions. The greater the number of possibilities, and the more unlike their outcomes, the more difficult it is to use the intuitive process of everyday life. Further, when the decision is not just a personal one, it is important to reach some agreement on how different outcomes should be valued. Agreements and disagreements are easier to spot if the valuing process is explicit.

At the workshop Kaplan described a method for valuing and summarizing health effects that has been developed to allow the comparison of interventions with very different health outcomes.[5] While the method has been applied to situations in which all changes in health are of interest, whether or not they affect work capacity, it could be adapted to value changes in work capacity.

As noted in chapter 2, the method depends on the notion that people can value different states of health on a scale that ranges from zero, for death, to 1.0, for optimum health. A state of disability that caused some discomfort and limited the individual's mobility might be valued at .59 compared with optimum health. A more severe state of disability that confined the sufferer to bed might be valued at only .34 as good as optimum health. Once different states of health are assigned values on the same scale, it becomes possible to combine them into an overall measure of health that summarizes the effects of an intervention.

An example will illustrate how the method works. Consider an individual who lives for 71.6 years. During 65.2 of those years he is completely well. During the next 4.5 years he suffers from disabilities that do not confine him to bed, and during the final 1.9 years he is confined to bed. With the values from the preceding paragraph, it is possible to calculate the value of these successive health states in an equivalent number of years of optimum health, called "well-years" for short. The first 65.2 years are valued at 1.0, because they are years of optimum health. The next 4.5 years are valued at .59 and the final 1.9 years at .34. The results are then added to arrive at the number of well years:

$$
\begin{aligned}
65.2 \times 1.0 &= 65.2 \\
4.5 \times .59 &= 2.7 \\
1.9 \times .34 &= \underline{.6} \\
&\ 68.5
\end{aligned}
$$

Thus the 71.6 years of life are equivalent to 68.5 well-years because the quality of life during the later years is reduced by disability and ill health.

Now suppose that a preventive intervention is applied that eliminates the first stage of disability. These years are now valued at 1.0 rather than .59 and the equivalent number of well-years rises to 70.3. The intervention receives credit for the difference of 1.8 well-years (70.3–68.5). Sup-

5. For a fuller description of the method, see Kaplan and Bush 1982. The model builds on the work reported in Fanshel and Bush 1970; Bush, Chen, and Patrick 1973; and Chen, Bush, and Patrick 1975.

Table 3-1. *Function Classification*

Mobility
  Drove car and used bus or train without help
  Did not drive, or had help to use bus or train
  In house
  In hospital
  In special care unit
Physical activity
  Walked without physical problems
  Walked with physical limitations
  Moved own wheelchair without help
  In bed or chair
Social Activity
  Did work, school, or housework and other activities
  Did work, school, or housework but other activities limited
  Limited in amount or kind of work, school, or housework
  Performed self-care but not work, school, or housework
  Had help with self-care

Source: Kaplan and Bush 1982.

pose that a second intervention makes it possible to eliminate the period of bed confinement so that the entire life span is one of good health. The second intervention then receives credit for 1.3 well-years (71.6–70.3). The common unit—well-years—makes it possible to summarize different states of health in a single measure and thus to compare two interventions with different outcomes.

To put the idea into practice, the researchers who developed this approach had to develop methods for assigning values to states of health. Different diseases can produce similar effects and symptoms so they focused on the effects and symptoms rather than on diseases. They began by identifying the important ways in which poor health could affect an individual. They organized these effects into three scales—mobility, physical activity, and social activity—and a list of "symptom/problem complexes." The items in each of the three scales are shown in table 3-1. There are twenty-one separate symptom and problem complexes ranging from none, to wearing eyeglasses, to spells of feeling upset, being depressed, or crying, to extensive burns.

Any particular state of health is a combination of elements from the three scales and the symptom/problem complexes. To find out how people value the separate elements the researchers surveyed a random sample of more than 800 people in their local community, San Diego, California. The respondents were presented with a series of cases describing states of health and were asked to assign a value to each case. The elements making up each case were changed in a systematic pattern from one case to the next. Using regression analysis, the researchers were able to relate the overall values and the elements to arrive at individual values for each element.[6]

The researchers have put the method to a number of tests. For example, in a study of patients with chronic obstructive lung disease they found that health status as measured on the well-year scale correlated best with the best single measure of lung function.[7] They point out that the two should not be perfectly correlated because the health status measure is a more comprehensive measure of health than the lung function test. Another study tested the assumption, implicit in the method, that a particular symptom or function makes the same difference to the overall level of health regardless of the other symptoms and functions with which it is combined.[8] Analysis of individuals' ratings of different states of overall health supported the assumption.[9]

The method has been used in several cost-effectiveness studies. It permits investigators to calculate the gain from an intervention in terms of well-years, compare these with the costs, and then compare the cost per well-year gained of alternative interventions. The method has been used to evaluate a program of screening and treatment for intestinal parasites in Indochinese refugees to the United States,[10] a program of screening and treatment for phenylketonuria in newborns,[11] a program of rehabilitative treatment for patients with chronic obstructive lung disease,[12] and programs to follow up abnormal results on screening blood tests.[13]

For these applications and others, the advantage of the method is that it allows a wide variety of health effects to be expressed in a common unit, the well-year, and compared. Both good and bad health effects can be evaluated. For example, as Weinstein and Stason illustrated in their study

6. Kaplan, Bush, and Berry 1978.

7. Kaplan, Atkins, and Timms 1984.

8. Kaplan 1982.

9. Other tests of the reliability and validity of the model are reported in Kaplan, Bush, and Berry 1976; Kaplan, Bush, and Berry 1978; and Kaplan 1982.

10. Anderson and Moser 1985.

11. Bush, Chen, and Patrick 1973.

12. Atkins, Kaplan, Timms, and others 1984; Kaplan, Atkins, and Timms 1984; and Toevs, Kaplan, and Atkins 1984.

13. Epstein, Schneiderman, Bush, and others 1981; and Amberg, Schneiderman, Berry, and others 1982.

of hypertension, reductions in the quality of life because of side effects can be evaluated and subtracted from the gains in health brought by the intervention.

Kaplan emphasized the value of a health status index that is as general as possible and contrasted its use with the uses appropriate to measures specific to a particular disease or intervention. He pointed out, for example, that a clinical study to compare two different methods for rehabilitating patients with serious burns on their hands would want to focus on the patients' ability to manipulate their hands and fingers. A specific index to measure that aspect of functioning is appropriate in that situation even though it then becomes impossible to compare the results of that intervention with, say, a program to help people quit smoking.

For policy purposes, however, it is necessary to have a measure of health effects—like the well-year—that is not specific to a particular disease or intervention, but that captures the important consequences of all of them. Kaplan emphasized that the ideal measure would incorporate mental as well as physical health and would permit health to be measured at any stage during the life cycle, from childhood to old age. He noted, for example, that separate measures for adults and children would make it difficult to evaluate some preventive measures, such as childhood vaccinations that continue to protect, and thus to produce health benefits, during adulthood. He noted that all health providers are attempting to improve the quality of life and extend its duration. It is valuable to allow them to use a common unit to compare the benefits of their services.

What Remains to Be Done

Both discussants agreed that the weak part of the methods proposed for translating health effects into capacity to work, or even for valuing more general health effects, is the estimation of time spent in each state of disability. Not much work has gone into this part of the methodology and the assumptions generally made are that health is stable over long periods of time or that it deteriorates steadily and in a linear fashion. Marilyn Bergner gave some examples where this is clearly not the case. Alzheimer's disease often proceeds slowly at first, then rapidly for a while, and then reaches a plateau where any further deterioration is minor. The health effects of arthritis, by contrast, fluctuate widely over a short period, even during a single day. Measures of capacity to work taken at one or a few points during the period of disability could seriously misrepresent capacity to work over the whole period. Thus the problem is both to measure the time spent in any given state and to measure all important changes in state.

Kaplan suggested that it would not be difficult to include measures of the duration of disability in prospective studies and that some of the fluctuations in the capacity of individuals would average out when groups of people were considered. More generally, Michele C. Adler asked that analysts involved in planning federal surveys consider incorporating questions that would help fill in some of the missing links, such as the pattern of disability over time, and test some of the standard concepts, such as the activities of daily living.

Bergner observed that, in its current form, the well-year does not distinguish between gains in health that affect capacity to work and those that do not. It needs adaptation before it can be used to value different states of work capacity. She suggested that some of the elements already part of the well-year method lend themselves to an adapted version and that other, existing information could help, such as the data on the relation between work and specific diseases collected by the Rand Corporation as part of the Health Insurance Experiment.[14]

Patrick noted the omission of mental health from the methods linking disease to disability, and, to some extent, from the well-year. The omission is important because mental disorders are a leading reason people qualify for government disability benefits.[15] He also stressed the need for further testing of the assumptions behind the methods presented, to check that they accurately reflect clinical and epidemiological knowledge about disability. He stressed the value of a method like the well-year for representing the net effects of simultaneous risk factors and interventions. Risk factors and diseases are combined in complicated ways and models of health effects need to reflect the interrelationships.

He returned to the distinction between ability to work and willingness to work. For some people, the only kinds of work for which they are qualified are onerous, increasingly so as they grow older—heavy manual labor is an example. He reminded the participants that these people might choose to stop working even if improvements in health made it possible for them to continue.

14. Avery, Lelah, Solomon, and others 1976. This report describes the plan to collect such data. The data were subsequently collected but have not been analyzed.

15. U.S. Senate, Special Committee on Aging 1984.

part two   **Assessing the Evidence**

George A. Bray
Virginia L. Ernster
Donald W. Goodwin
Thomas A. Hodgson
John H. Holbrook
Harold D. Holder
Gerry Oster
William A. Peck
Kenneth E. Powell
Richard S. Rivlin
David Siscovick
Jane E. Sisk
Albert J. Stunkard
Ernestine Vanderveen
Brian T. Yates

At the workshop participants reviewed the epidemio-
logical and medical evidence in five areas besides hypertension—smoking,
exercise, dietary calcium, alcohol use, and obesity—to assess whether
that evidence is good enough to support cost-effectiveness analyses. The
primary focus of the review was on the adverse health effects of smoking,
lack of exercise, and so on, and on the evidence that changing behavior
avoids or reverses those effects. Although they were not asked to spend
much time on the effectiveness of specific interventions, or their costs, the
participants contributed a good deal of information about these subjects as
well.

In each session the author of the background paper began by reviewing
the medical and epidemiological evidence. One of the discussants was an
epidemiologist or physician; the other was a researcher familiar with cost-
effectiveness analysis. The discussants' task was to engage the author and
each other in a conversation about the evidence, as if they were planning
to undertake a cost-effectiveness analysis together.

Each session covered much of the preliminary work necessary for an
analysis, providing not only the foundation on which to judge its feasibility
but also many of the elements essential to it. The summaries do not follow
the chronological order of the presentations but weave them together to
reflect better the pattern that emerged.

chapter four **Smoking**

Rarely has any area been so thoroughly studied as smoking. There is so much information, of such good quality, that there can be no question about the feasibility of a cost-effectiveness evaluation. Rather the questions have to do with how best to make use of the information and how to deal with the inevitable problems of combining information from different sources and using historical data to model the future. The participants indicated that in several areas data are available that have not been fully exploited for what they can show about important relationships between, for example, smoking and disability, or between certain kinds of antismoking interventions and their costs and effects.

Health Effects

John H. Holbrook succinctly reviewed the voluminous evidence on health effects. He began by identifying the largest prospective epidemiological studies—studies that tracked large numbers of people over many years to determine the effects of smoking.[1] Four of the eight studies were done in the United States, and one each in Britain, Japan, Canada, and Sweden. While the studies tended to concentrate on men, three of them—

John H. Holbrook wrote and presented the background paper. *Thomas A. Hodgson* and *Virginia L. Ernster* were the discussants.

1. These studies were reviewed in U.S. Public Health Service 1979. The original citations for each study are provided in the rest of this footnote, with all those for one study separated by a period from those for the next study. Doll and Hill 1956, 1964a, 1964b, 1966; Doll and Peto 1976 and 1977. Hammond 1965, 1966, 1972; Hammond and Garfinkel 1969; and Hammond, Garfinkel, Seidman, and others 1976. Dorn 1958; Kahn 1966; Rogot 1974a and 1974b. Hirayama 1967, 1970, 1972, and 1975. Best, Josie, and Walker 1961; and Canadian Department of National Health and Welfare 1966. Hammond and Horn 1958. Dunn, Jr., Linden, and Breslow 1960; Weir and Dunn, Jr., 1970; and Cederlof, Friberg, Hrubec, and Lorich 1975.

one U.S. study, and the Japanese and Swedish studies—included large numbers of women.[2]

Taken together the studies show that, for men, the death rate for smokers is about 70 percent higher than the death rate for nonsmokers. This figure lumps all smokers together. When smokers are distinguished by how much they smoke, the risk of death rises steadily with the number of cigarettes. For those who smoke less than half a pack a day, death rates are 30 percent to 40 percent higher than those of nonsmokers. For two-pack-a-day smokers the death rate is approximately double that of nonsmokers.[3]

Cardiovascular disease, cancer, and bronchitis and emphysema are the major causes of the extra deaths among smokers, but the adverse effects of smoking extend well beyond those three categories of disease.[4] To underscore this point, Holbrook showed that smoking is associated with a higher risk of death from nearly all of the ten leading causes of death in the United States, from heart disease to accidents to influenza and pneumonia. In a few cases it is not yet clear whether the relationship is one of cause and effect—it may sometimes be due, or due in part, to other differences between smokers and nonsmokers.

The impact of smoking on deaths from particular causes can be calculated in terms of "attributable risk"—the proportion of deaths attributed to smoking. The Office of Technology Assessment estimates that, in 1982, 32 percent of all cancer deaths, 13 percent of all deaths from cardiovascular disease, and 88 percent of all deaths from chronic lung disease were due to smoking—a total of more than 300,000 deaths from these three causes alone.[5]

Smoking is associated with more illness and disability than not smoking. Smokers, particularly younger smokers, are somewhat more likely to suffer from chronic conditions, often the same ones that lead to their higher death rates. There is some indication that smokers are more often limited in their activities by chronic conditions than nonsmokers, although the pattern is not consistent, possibly because the data do not distinguish light smokers from heavy ones. A more consistent finding is that smokers lose more days from work each year than nonsmokers.[6]

2. The U.S. study is the American Cancer Society study reported in the publications by Hammond and others cited in footnote 1.
3. U.S. Public Health Service 1979.
4. Kuller 1982.
5. Office of Technology Assessment 1985.
6. U.S. Public Health Service 1981.

The list of adverse health effects grows with every new study. Smokers suffer from peptic ulcers more often than nonsmokers do. They develop complications after surgery more frequently. Dental problems, periodontal disease, and infertility are all more common in smokers. Nor are the effects limited to the smokers themselves. Pregnant women who smoke have more stillbirths and their babies are smaller on average, more likely to die soon after birth, and more likely to experience problems with physical and intellectual development as they grow up. Evidence is increasing that "passive smoking" has ill effects on the health of nonsmokers, both children and adults.[7]

Research has documented in considerable detail the connection between the amount of exposure to smoking and its adverse effects—the "dose-response" relationship. This is an important element not only in establishing causation between smoking and disease, but in modeling the link for cost-effectiveness analysis. The risk of death and disease rises steadily the more cigarettes the individual smokes per day and the longer he or she smokes. For example, men who have smoked for less than fifteen years have a death rate about 10 percent higher than nonsmokers, while those who have smoked for thirty-five years or more have a death rate that is 66 percent higher.[8] Not everyone reacts to smoking the same way, however—some people never suffer serious adverse effects—and the reasons for the differences are not yet well understood. In some cases, exposure to air pollution on the job reinforces the harm done by smoking, or smoking interacts with drugs (the contraceptive pill, for example), but in other cases the differences appear to be because of genetic or other factors not yet identified.

For capacity to work, the data on illness and disability associated with smoking are particularly important. Lowering the death rate would lengthen the work life of many people, but reducing illness and disability affects their capacity for work during years that would be lived anyway as well as during added years. Statistics on days lost from work show that, for men, those who have ever smoked—both current and former smokers—lose one or two more days from work each year than nonsmokers. Among younger women, current smokers lose about a day more a year than nonsmokers, but there are no differences between former smokers and nonsmokers, or among older women regardless of their smoking

7. Holbrook 1987.
8. U.S. Public Health Service 1979.

habits. Since these data do not distinguish among smokers according to the amount they smoke, or did smoke, they may disguise stronger relationships for heavy smokers (the lesser effect for women most likely reflects the fact that, until recently, they generally smoked less than men). Nonetheless, the data show that smoking, even crudely measured, has a significant impact on the working capacity of younger adults and on older men nearing or in retirement.

Interventions

Interventions can be directed at helping current smokers quit, to prevent or reduce adverse health effects, or at persuading nonsmokers not to start. The statistics already reviewed on the health of smokers compared with nonsmokers show clearly that it is preferable not to start smoking.

It has also been established beyond question that quitting is beneficial.[9] Studies have tracked smokers who quit to find out how long it takes the benefits to show up and how great the benefits are. Some benefits appear almost immediately, while others take years to appear, and some adverse effects cannot be reversed. Deaths from heart disease begin to decline sharply within months after a smoker quits. In contrast, the damage to the lungs is often irreversible, and the best the exsmoker can hope for is to lose lung function no faster than a nonsmoker, starting from the lower level established by smoking.

When all diseases are considered, those who smoked less than a pack a day return to the death rates of nonsmokers ten years after they quit. Heavier smokers still show higher death rates at ten years, but the rates decline from double the nonsmokers' rate in the first year after quitting to about one-third higher at ten years. In fact, in the first year after quitting, heavy smokers may have higher death rates than smokers of the same age, possibly because they quit in response to serious health problems.

Quitting has adverse side effects, as any former smoker will attest. They may include a modest weight gain, the difficulty of giving up an addictive behavior—which involves withdrawal symptoms in the early stages, and the need to find some replacement behavior for the situations in which the smoker particularly turned to smoking. If there are side

9. Hammond 1965; and the 1982, 1983, and 1984 Surgeon General's Reports of the U.S. Public Health Service. Studies of British physicians and young American men found that, in both groups, substantial declines in smoking were followed by substantial declines in lung cancer rates. Doll and Peto 1976; and Winkelstein, Jr., 1985.

effects to interventions that keep people from smoking in the first place, no one suggested what they are.

The specific intervention that probably comes first to mind is a special program, or perhaps counseling by a physician, to help smokers quit. Many people have also heard of nicotine chewing gum, which helps smokers get through the first difficult weeks of withdrawal. If a second intervention comes to mind, it is likely to be school programs to educate children and adolescents about smoking and help them avoid becoming smokers in the first place. The vast majority of people who smoke begin as teenagers. Holbrook mentioned that there are some very promising models for school programs.

Virginia L. Ernster stressed that the possible interventions cover a much wider range than counseling and school education. Interventions begin with the research that documents the harmful effects of smoking and the benefits of quitting. Without that research the subsequent steps that have so dramatically changed public attitudes toward smoking in the last thirty years would not have been possible. These steps include widespread dissemination of research findings through government reports and the media, public service advertisements against smoking, restrictions on the advertising of cigarettes, and informational brochures in physicians' offices. They include laws restricting smoking in the workplace and other public places and the informal arrangements by which restaurants and hotels, for example, have set up smoking and nonsmoking areas to accommodate the preferences of their customers.

At least some of these measures, perhaps all, have been effective in some degree—the proportion of men who smoke dropped from about half in the 1950s to about one-third today.[10] But the costs and effectiveness of alternative interventions have not been carefully studied. Most of the evaluations that have been done have focused on smoking cessation programs, which are the easiest intervention to study, but which reach relatively few people. They are not, of course, directed at people who have not yet started to smoke but may be thinking of it, and they reach only a few smokers—about 95 percent of those who quit do so on their own, without formal help.[11] Very little is known about the costs and effects of more general interventions, such as school programs, public service ad-

10. The proportion of women who smoke has shown little change; in fact, the proportion of *young* women who smoke has risen in recent years.

11. It is not known how many of these people may have tried special programs or counseling in earlier attempts to quit. People who succeed in quitting generally try several times before they are successful.

vertising, or laws restricting smoking. Henry Blackburn suggested that data are now available from research demonstrations in Minnesota and elsewhere that could be used to evaluate these interventions.

Other possible interventions have not yet been used explicitly against smoking. Excise taxes could be raised and the higher price of cigarettes would discourage smoking. Restrictions could be placed on the distribution and sale of cigarettes, similar to the restrictions on the sale of alcoholic beverages. All advertising of cigarettes could be banned. Programs could be created to encourage tobacco farmers to get out of the business.

The interventions with the greatest short-term impact on capacity to work are probably those that help current smokers quit. Since most smokers do quit on their own, general forces such as advertising and the warnings of friends, family, and physicians, backed up by research, may be as important as more specific aids like smoking cessation programs or nicotine chewing gum. More general interventions aimed at keeping people from beginning to smoke would have their effects over a longer period of time.

Cost-Effectiveness Analysis

Thomas A. Hodgson outlined the data that might be used to model health effects for a cost-effectiveness analysis. He suggested that the American Cancer Society study would be a good basis for modeling the death rates from smoking.[12] This study was not based on a representative sample, but the relationships derived from it could be applied to estimates of population by age, sex, and smoking status based on the National Health Interview Study, which is a representative sample.

The illness and disability caused by smoking have not yet been as carefully documented as its effects on life expectancy. Much remains to be learned about the impact of smoking on functional capacity, the length of time smokers suffer impaired health, and the quality of life during that time. Hodgson suggested two sources of data that contain a great deal of information about the illness and disability caused by smoking and that have not yet been exploited for all they can tell. One is the National Health Interview Survey, which has been conducted annually since 1957 and

12. See Hammond 1965, 1966, and 1972; Hammond and Garfinkel 1969; and Hammond, Garfinkel, Seidman, and others 1976.

which includes questions on smoking from time to time beginning in the 1964–65 period. The other is the National Health and Nutrition Examination Survey, and the Epidemiological Follow-up Survey, which conducted physical examinations of a sample of 14,000 people in the 1971–75 period and in the 1982–83 and 1986–87 periods.[13]

Even in the area of smoking, with its rich array of studies, the range of uncertainty is surprisingly large. Although the link between smoking and mortality is thoroughly documented, estimates of the deaths attributable to smoking vary by a factor of two around the number produced by the Office of Technology Assessment. The uncertainty is increased because a cost-effectiveness analysis is concerned with projecting the future effects of current smoking patterns, while the data pertain to the current effects of past smoking. Smoking patterns are changing, the nature of cigarettes is changing, and other factors that affect health are changing. These changes will require judgment in the use of historical data to create a model of health effects and the liberal use of sensitivity analyses to test the importance of alternative assumptions.

13. See, for example, U.S. National Center for Health Statistics 1986.

chapter five   Exercise

The term exercise covers a wide diversity of activities, from jogging to competitive sports to specific movements designed to stretch or strengthen a particular muscle. Its effects can be expected to be equally diverse. Studies have examined a number of these possible effects, often without defining the nature of the exercise precisely. Indeed, most studies have not examined exercise specifically—that is, activity directed at improving physical fitness—but physical activity more broadly, including such things as activity on the job; the session participants urged that the two terms be kept distinct and not used interchangeably.[1] The subject that has received the most attention is the effect of aerobic activity, which conditions the heart and lungs, on coronary heart disease.

Health Effects

David Siscovick began by reviewing the evidence linking physical activity to lower rates of heart disease. Three major studies have tracked the experience of large numbers of middle-aged men over a decade or more. One looked at the activity on the job of San Francisco longshoremen,[2] another at the leisure activity of British civil servants,[3] and the third at the leisure activity of Harvard alumni.[4] All three found that men who engaged in vigorous physical activity experienced lower death rates from heart attack and lower rates of nonfatal heart disease as well. For deaths, the rate for men who engaged in vigorous activity was approximately half the

David Siscovick wrote and presented the background paper. *Jane E. Sisk* and *Kenneth E. Powell* were the discussants.

1. Caspersen, Powell, and Christenson 1985.
2. Paffenbarger and Hale 1975; and Brand, Paffenbarger, Jr., Scholtz, and Kampert 1979.
3. Morris, Everitt, Pollard, and Chave 1980; and Morris, Everitt, Pollard and others 1981.
4. Paffenbarger, Jr., Wing, and Hyde 1978.

rate for those who did not. Several smaller studies have produced the same result.[5]

None of the studies randomly assigned some men to vigorous activity and others to inactivity. The men being studied had made their own decisions about how much activity to engage in, or had the decision made for them by their jobs, and the researchers simply observed the differences between those who did more and those who did less. Because of this it is possible that the results reflect "selection, not protection"—that people who are healthier are more likely to be active rather than that physical activity makes people healthier.

Researchers have used several strategies to try to determine whether the relationship is truly one of cause and effect. In each study the population selected was free of heart disease at the outset; thus disease did not cause the initial differences in activity. Each study also collected information on other factors that might be related to heart disease—smoking, hypertension, weight, a family history of heart disease, and the like, and corrected for those factors in the analysis; in every case activity was associated with lower rates of coronary deaths even after the correction.[6] The Harvard Alumni study checked the possibility that an individual's inherited constitution controlled the outcome by comparing men who had been varsity athletes in college with those who had not been. College athletics turned out to have no connection with later heart attacks, but current activity did.

That regular physical activity protects against heart disease overall does not rule out the possibility that the risk of a heart attack may be transiently higher during activity itself. A study of men in Seattle found that heart attacks did in fact occur more frequently during vigorous activity—the rate was higher than the average rate for sedentary people during the same length of time—but that the protective effect of activity outweighed this transiently higher risk.[7] Thus the stories of people dying suddenly during strenuous activity are consistent with the finding that activity is associated with a lower rate of heart attack overall.

The study of Harvard alumni also examined deaths from all causes and found that the more active men had lower death rates.[8] The major reason for the difference was, of course, fewer deaths from heart disease, but the

5. Siscovick, Weiss, Hallstrom, and others 1982; Garcia-Palmieri, Costas, Cruz-Vidal, and others 1982; and Salonen, Puska, and Tuomilehto 1982.

6. Cholesterol level was not measured except in the study of British civil servants.

7. Siscovick, Weiss, Fletcher, and others 1984.

8. Paffenbarger, Jr., Hyde, and Wing 1986.

result confirms that physical activity promotes long life in general and that its good effects on heart disease are not offset by harmful effects on other diseases. Again, these results held even after correction for the other factors that might have affected the men's health.

Other research suggests that regular physical activity has beneficial effects on many diseases besides heart disease. Observational studies— studies that, like those of heart disease, simply observe differences between people who are more active and those who are less—show that vigorous physical activity may reduce the risk of developing high blood pressure. Their results are reinforced by clinical studies showing that exercise helps control hypertension once it develops. The research on the subject is not entirely in agreement, however, possibly because of small samples, the diversity of physical activity, or other differences in the populations studied.[9] Similarly, epidemiological studies, clinical observation, and small clinical trials suggest that regular physical activity may help prevent or control noninsulin dependent diabetes and osteoporosis.[10] In both cases, however, activity poses potential risks that have not been fully investigated—adverse diabetic reactions have been reported after exercise and fractures during exercise might offset the gains for osteoporosis.

The effects of physical activity on ability to function and well-being have not been as thoroughly studied as its effects on heart disease or longevity, but there are strong indications of potentially important benefits. These benefits are particularly important for capacity to work. For example, regular vigorous activity improves the capacity to perform physical work.[11] Over periods of eight hours or longer people can work at only 20 percent to 25 percent of their maximum capacity, and when that capacity is low, fatigue can become a chronic problem.[12] By increasing the

9. Hicky, Mulcahy, Bourke, and others 1975; Cooper, Pollock, Martin, and others 1976; Gibbons, Blair, Cooper, and others 1983; Boyer and Kasch 1970; Choquette and Ferguson 1973; Kukkonen, Rauramaa, Voutilainen, and others 1982; Duncan, Farr, Upton, and others 1985; Roman, Camuzzi, Villalon, and Klenner 1981; Paffenbarger, Jr., Wing, Hyde, and Jung 1983; and Blair, Goodyear, Gibbons, and Cooper 1984.

10. On diabetes, see Richter, Ruderman, and Schneider 1981; King, Taylor, Zimmet, and others 1984; and Zimmet, Faaiuso, Ainuu, and others 1981. On osteoporosis, see Chalmers and Ho 1970; Aloia, Cohn, Babu, and others 1978; Dalén and Olsson 1974; Krølner, Toft, Nielsen, and others 1983; Aloia 1981; Stein, Sabato, Leichter, and others 1983; Krølner and Toft 1983; Hansson, Roos, and Nachemson 1975; Whedon and Shorr 1957; Freedman 1949; Mazess and Whedon 1983; and Drinkwater, Nilson, Chesnut III, and others 1984.

11. Shephard, Cox, and Corey 1981; Linden 1969.

12. Haskell and Blair 1980.

capacity for physical work, exercise helps reduce fatigue and could improve older people's ability to hold jobs. The results for hypertension, diabetes, and osteoporosis are also relevant for work capacity since all three conditions can cause disability.

In addition, clinical observation and research studies indicate that exercise improves mood and helps combat depression and anxiety, effects that could improve people's capacity for work.[13] The Stanford Heart Disease Program, in which people were randomly assigned to exercise a little, a lot, or not at all, found that depression declined most among those who exercised most.[14]

Siscovick focused his review on the conditions that have been studied most thoroughly, but he noted that the complete list is much longer. Research has indicated that regular physical activity may affect obesity, peripheral vascular disease, stroke, lipid disorders, chronic lung disease, asthma, and cancer. The results in these areas are less definitive than in the areas reviewed.

The available research also gives some information about the dose-response relationship between activity and its effects, particularly for heart disease. That information does not define the type of activity precisely but measures it in terms of the energy expended. The study of Harvard alumni estimated the kilocalories (calories in lay language) used for walking, stair climbing, and sports. Death rates from all causes declined steadily as energy expenditure increased from 500 kilocalories to 3,500 kilocalories a week. For energy expenditures above 3,500 kilocalories death rates rose slightly, indicating that more activity was not beneficial beyond that point and might be harmful.[15]

Interventions

The studies of large populations have not attempted to change people's behavior, that is, to get people to take up exercise. Without randomly assigning people to exercise or not—which means that some who do not exercise now would have to, and some who do would have to stop—it is not possible to be sure that the benefits that have been observed are entirely because of physical activity. While this leaves some question

13. Taylor, Sallis, and Needle 1985.
14. William Haskell, personal communication to Albert J. Stunkard.
15. Paffenbarger, Jr., Hyde, and Wing 1986.

about the size of the benefit that would result from persuading people to exercise, the participants were persuaded that most people would benefit. The evidence is consistent in showing that physical activity confers benefits, that the effects are specific to activity and independent of other factors, and that they are related to the amount of activity.

Thus the evidence supports intervening to persuade people to exercise, particularly men, who have been the subjects in the major studies. The unresolved issues have to do with the benefits, risks, and costs of different kinds of exercise for different individuals. The results of the Harvard study notwithstanding, much remains to be learned about the type, intensity, frequency, and duration of activity necessary to achieve particular benefits and minimize risks. It is important to learn more about the exercise appropriate to each stage of life, from childhood to old age. While exercise can be used therapeutically—programs have been developed, for example, for people who have chronic lung disease or who have had a heart attack—the discussion concentrated on the kinds of exercise that could be recommended for large groups of people, most of them in good health.

Some people seem to benefit more than others from exercise and some may not benefit at all. Interventions should be tailored carefully to help those who can gain and avoid hurting those who cannot. Several of the heart disease studies suggest, for example, that the benefits of activity are greatest for people over 60 years of age, those with high blood pressure, and those who are overweight.[16] The study of mortality from all causes also shows greater benefit for older people and those with hypertension.[17] At the same time, results from a major trial of drugs to lower cholesterol indicate that men with very high cholesterol levels—265 milligrams per deciliter or higher—may not benefit from activity; in this group vigorous activity was not related to the risk of death from heart disease.[18] The Seven Countries study also shows that people with severe hypercholesterolemia do not benefit from higher levels of activity.

The findings for older people are particularly interesting for the evaluation of the capacity to work and suggest the value of research to learn more about the benefits and risks of exercise for older people. Henry Blackburn observed that low-intensity exercise, whose value has been studied rela-

16. Morris, Everitt, Pollard, and Chave 1980; Paffenbarger, Jr., Wing, and Hyde 1978; Paffenbarger, Jr., Hyde, Wing, and Steinmetz 1984; and Siscovick, Weiss, Fletcher, and others 1984.
17. Paffenbarger, Jr., Hyde, and Wing 1986.
18. David Siscovick, personal communication.

tively little, is the only feasible kind for most older people because their capacity has declined. How much of the decline in capacity with age is inevitable and how much is simply due to disuse is not entirely clear. Several reports suggest, however, that regular vigorous activity maintains the physical work capacity of aging adults, or at least slows its decline.[19]

Siscovick suggested that the more easily physical activity can be incorporated into people's lives, the more readily they will take it up, and that more attention should be given to developing exercise programs that become a natural extension of everyday activities. A study of children compared two approaches, one that engaged children in "programmed" sports and one that integrated exercise into their daily lives, for example, by encouraging them to do more walking and stair climbing. At the end of the study the results were the same for both groups, but when the researchers checked back a year later, they found that the children in the programmed sports group had returned to their earlier habits, while those in the group that had been encouraged to exercise in ways that fit in with their usual lives had continued the new habits and continued to benefit from exercise.[20]

Siscovick was concerned, however, that the risks of exercise, its "side effects," have not been well documented. A few good studies have examined the risks connected with running—Kenneth E. Powell cited a study showing that besides the risk of sprains and strains, runners are sometimes bitten by dogs or hit by cars or bicycles.[21] But there is little or nothing about other forms of exercise, and even with running, nothing is known about its longer-term effects. He stressed the importance of not assuming that the benefits outweigh the risks, particularly for certain groups for which the benefits may be small. Injuries have an impact on capacity to work as well. One participant suggested that the National Health Interview Survey might provide data that could show the risks of exercise for a general population.[22]

19. Åstrand 1960; Heath, Hagberg, Ehsani, and Holloszy 1981; Dehn and Bruce 1972; and Grimby and Saltin, 1966.

20. Epstein, Wing, Koeske, and others 1982.

21. Koplan, Powell, Sikes, and others 1982. See also Lane, Bloch, Jones, and others 1986; Panush, Schmidt, Caldwell, and others 1986; and Powell, Kohl, Caspersen, and Blair 1986.

22. Gerry Oster cited studies showing that preventive programs, like exercise, may induce people to use more medical care because, although they are healthier, they are also more aware of health problems and more inclined to seek advice. He asked whether that should be counted as an adverse side effect of a program.

In general, the costs of exercise include special equipment and clothing, facilities, leaders if these are required, and the costs of treating side effects. Clearly, these cannot be estimated without a fairly specific idea of the type of exercise program and the likely rate of injuries. More generally, not much is known about the costs of persuading people to take up exercise. The point from the smoking session applies here as well. Intervention includes more than the specific program of exercise; it includes the communitywide or nationwide flows of research and information that begin to persuade people to think seriously about changing their habits.

Cost-Effectiveness Analysis

Exercise differs from other forms of prevention in two important respects. It takes considerable time: Powell calculated that running twenty miles each week requires an average of twenty-eight minutes a day. On the other hand, many people derive pleasure simply from the exercise itself. Consider the contrast with antihypertensive medication or a vaccination. Neither takes very much time and neither gives any pleasure in and of itself. In fact, most people dislike taking pills or getting shots. Thus time is an important cost for exercise and pleasure—for some people at least—is an important benefit. The pleasure would not be relevant to an evaluation that focuses on capacity to work, but it may be relevant to a more comprehensive evaluation of the effects of exercise, and certainly to the individual's own evaluation of it. Several participants warned against assuming, however, that everyone does or would derive pleasure from exercise, just as not everyone shares the same tastes in other activities.

Powell argued that it makes no sense to evaluate exercise as a whole since it comes in so many forms and has so many different effects. In keeping with this view, several specific cost-effectiveness studies were proposed.

Jane E. Sisk suggested that there is adequate information to support an evaluation of the effects of exercise on heart disease. Good data show the rates of heart disease and the trends in those rates for the population. The studies reviewed by Siscovick show the size of the benefits, the relationship between the amount of physical activity and benefits, and even some detail on the differences among subgroups. Although data on the risks of exercise are harder to come by, there are the studies of runners, including elderly runners. She noted that it is not clear whether the findings for men apply to women or to minorities of either sex and that the studies show little about health gains in addition to lower death rates, but assumptions could be made about these elements of the model and tested through sensitivity analysis. This kind of evaluation would produce an estimate of benefits that could be viewed as a minimum because it would omit any beneficial effects of exercise on other conditions.

Powell suggested that enough is known to evaluate the effects of running twenty miles a week for men aged 30 to 64. Here again, he suggested that the modeling of benefits may have to be limited to heart disease because the evidence for other benefits is not yet good enough.

Powell also suggested that other specific evaluations might be undertaken with the idea that they could suggest which missing items of information were most important; the results would identify areas of high priority for research.

Exercise offers a particularly good example of the need to begin looking at all the health effects of an intervention, not just its effects on a single disease. It might be possible to build models of health effects based on the available evidence that would suggest the overall picture. But epidemiological and medical studies should also begin to take a more comprehensive view of the effects of physical activity, and to look not only at mortality from all causes but at illness, ability to function, and mental health in the same study. Robert M. Kaplan pointed out that a method like the well-year would allow all the effects of exercise, physical and mental, to be incorporated in a single summary measure.

chapter six   **Dietary Calcium**

The reason for the current interest in dietary calcium is that it may help prevent osteoporosis, a condition in which an individual's bone mass is too low to withstand even minor injury without fracturing.[1] In 1984 a Consensus Conference convened by the National Institutes of Health to review the prevention and treatment of osteoporosis recommended that adults get 1,000 milligrams of calcium a day, except for women past menopause and not receiving estrogen replacement therapy, who should consume 1,500 milligrams;[2] both amounts are higher than the Recommended Dietary Allowance of 800 milligrams for adults.

The discussion at the workshop focused on the evidence that calcium is effective in preventing osteoporosis; that evidence is still less complete and convincing than many experts would like. Concerns were also expressed about whether it makes sense to recommend a single nutrient as the solution for a single condition when there are so many interactions among nutrients and among conditions.

Health Effects

At the outset of his review, William A. Peck noted that osteoporosis is an important affliction because of the devastating consequences of the fractures that result from it. It causes about 1.3 million fractures every year, primarily of the wrist, hip, and spinal vertebrae. Wrist fractures, the least disabling, are very common, and hospitalization is required in 18 percent of the cases.[3] Vertebral fractures are the cause of Dowager's

William A. Peck wrote and presented the background paper. **Richard S. Rivlin** and **Gerry Oster** were the discussants.

1. Recent reviews are Cummings, Kelsey, Nevitt, and others 1985; Consensus Conference 1984; and Johnston, Jr., and Epstein 1981.
2. Consensus Conference 1984.
3. Alffram and Bauer 1962; and Owen, Melton III, Johnson, and others 1982.

hump, which afflicts approximately 500,000 people in the United States, most of them women. Multiple fractures of the spine can cause serious health problems and pain as the spine collapses and internal organs are compressed.[4]

Peck termed hip fractures the most serious consequence of osteoporosis.[5] Approximately 200,000 hip fractures occur every year. On average a hip fracture requires three weeks of hospitalization and the death rate for women in the following year is 6 percent to 11 percent among those less than 75 years old, and even higher in older women. More than half of the survivors lose their ability to live independently, and 25 percent to 35 percent become residents of nursing homes.

Half of all hip fractures occur in people under 80—almost one-third of this number in people under 65—and these have potentially important implications for work capacity. The other half occur in people over 80 years of age, people for whom the ability to work is unlikely to be an important issue although the ability to live independently certainly is.[6]

Most osteoporosis does not have a specific cause and is called "primary" osteoporosis. Bone mass increases until maturity, probably between 20 and 30 years of age for the trabecular bone that predominates in the spine and between 35 and 45 for the cortical bone that predominates in the arms and legs, and then declines thereafter as the individual ages.[7] Osteoporosis is the result of inadequate bone mass at maturity, excessive losses thereafter, or both, but why it occurs in some individuals, and not in others, is not known.

Some groups are, however, clearly at greater risk than others.[8] Osteoporosis is much more common in women than in men, in older people, in people who are thin, and in members of the Caucasian or Oriental races. Smoking, lack of exercise, and insufficient calcium are also associated with osteoporosis. In women bone loss accelerates during the period around menopause; apparently part of the reason is that the production of estrogen declines after menopause—estrogen deficiency is a recognized risk factor. Oral contraceptives, pregnancy, and estrogen replacement

4. Iskrant and Smith 1969; and Kleerekoper, Parfitt, and Ellis 1984.

5. Haupt and Graves 1982; Lewinnek, Kelsey, White, and others 1980; Weiss, Liff, Ure, and others 1983; and Keene and Anderson 1982.

6. Osteoporosis may also be an important cause of dental problems. See Wical and Brussee 1979.

7. Riggs, Wahner, Dunn, and others 1981.

8. Cummings, Kelsey, Nevitt, and others 1985; Consensus Conference 1984; and Johnston, Jr., 1985.

therapy all protect against osteoporosis—further evidence that estrogen deficiency may be a cause. Premature menopause, especially if induced by surgery, radiation, or certain chemotherapeutic drugs, puts a woman at greater risk.

Five of these risk factors offer potential points of intervention. Gaining weight is not usually an attractive possibility since most of the effects of overweight on health are undesirable. Smoking is, of course, undesirable on any ground, but some people continue to smoke. Estrogen replacement is a recognized therapy used for a number of women during and after menopause; it is, however, relatively expensive and its side effects are not well known. This leaves calcium supplementation and exercise, both of which appear promising as methods of populationwide intervention. The National Institutes of Health Consensus Conference recommended more weight-bearing exercise as well as higher levels of calcium.

Interventions

Many adult Americans do not get the Recommended Dietary Allowance of 800 milligrams of calcium a day, let alone the higher amounts recommended by the Consensus Conference.[9] One in four women consume less than 300 milligrams daily, and after the menopause the average woman consumes less than 600 milligrams a day. Between 1970 and 1980 calcium intake among teenagers declined significantly.

Several major lines of evidence support the idea that calcium intake is involved in osteoporosis. First, there are the facts about how calcium functions in the body. More than 99 percent of the body's calcium is stored in the bones. A very small amount circulates in the blood, where it is essential to the proper functioning of the organs. This circulating calcium must be maintained within a narrow range; when it is low, the bones release calcium, and when it is high, they may store the excess.[10] Certainly any significant changes in the overall amount of calcium in the body must be accompanied by significant changes in the amount of calcium in the bones. It can be demonstrated in laboratory tests that people lose calcium at the levels of intake common in the U.S. population. Small daily losses over a period of many years will be associated with a significant loss of bone tissue. Further, consistent with the fact that bone mass is lost as

9. Heaney 1985; Heaney, Gallagher, Johnston, and others 1982; and Heaney, Recker, and Saville 1977.
10. Heaney 1985.

people age, research has shown that the balance of calcium in the body deteriorates in women after the menopause,[11] and that calcium absorption and adaptation to calcium deprivation decline in older people.[12]

Epidemiological studies show that low calcium intake is associated with a higher incidence of osteoporosis, although they cannot separate low intake from the effect other nutrients may have by regulating the availability of the calcium to the body. Three studies are considered particularly good—Matkovic's study in Yugoslavia, Fujita's study in Japan, and Yano's study of Japanese residents in Hawaii[13]—and, of these, Peck cited Matkovic's study as providing the strongest evidence. In that study the populations in two areas of Yugoslavia, one with a high calcium intake and one with a low calcium intake, were compared. At every age from 30 onward, people in the high-calcium area had significantly greater appendicular bone mass than people in the low-calcium area; the effect of the calcium appeared to occur before the age of 30 and to persist with advancing age. More important, while the prevalence of hip fracture increased with age in both areas, it was much higher in the low-calcium area. The frequency of wrist fractures did not differ between the two areas.

The association is supported by other studies showing that active intervention to increase the amount of calcium people consume does appear to protect against osteoporosis.[14] The intervention studies suffer from various shortcomings—they are generally small, of short duration, and use intermediate measures of outcome, such as bone width or the balance of calcium in the body, rather than the outcome of fundamental interest, fractures; researchers are still not sure how close the link is between the intermediate measures and fractures. The studies have examined widely different populations, including healthy postmenopausal women and women already known to have osteoporosis. Nonetheless, several of them have found changes in these intermediate outcomes indicating that calcium can reduce osteoporosis.[15]

11. Heaney, Recker, and Saville 1977.

12. Bullamore, Gallagher, Wilkinson, and others 1970; Nordin, Wilkinson, Marshall, and others 1976; Gallagher, Riggs, Eisman, and others 1979; Avioli, McDonald, and Lee 1965; Ireland and Fordtran 1973; Alevizaki, Ikkos, and Singhelakis 1973; Parfitt, Gallagher, Heaney, and others 1982; Caniggia, Gennari, Bianchi, and others 1963; and Gallagher, Jerpbak, Jr., Jee, and others 1982.

13. Matkovic, Kostial, Simonovic, and others 1979; Fujita, Okamoto, Sakagami, and others 1984; and Yano, Heilbrun, Wasnich, and others 1985.

14. Thallassinos, Gutteridge, Joplin, and others 1982; Horowitz, Need, Philcox, and others 1984; Recker and Heaney 1985; and Riggs, Seeman, Hodgson, and others 1982.

15. The studies that produced less clear-cut results are: Recker, Saville, and Heaney

Several more specialized strands of evidence also support the link between calcium and osteoporosis. Lactose intolerance, a genetic sensitivity to milk, is common among Caucasians with osteoporosis.[16] A kidney condition, idiopathic renal hypercalciuria, in which abnormally large amounts of calcium are lost through the urine, is also associated with osteoporosis.[17] Thiazide diuretics, used to treat hypertension, reduce the excretion of calcium through the urine, and several studies have observed that they appear to protect bone.[18] Finally, experiments on animals have shown that severe calcium deprivation causes osteoporosis and that the osteoporosis can be cured when the animals are once again given enough calcium.[19]

Drawing primarily on the epidemiological studies, Peck concluded that while calcium helps determine bone mass, it is less important in this respect than race, age, sex, weight, height, or hormonal status. It probably has its greatest impact before the age of 30, and consumption must be adequate over long periods of time to be effective. He proposed that it would be optimistic to expect that optimal calcium intake would increase bone mass at maturity by even as much as 5 percent. Nonetheless, that might be enough to make a substantial difference in the rate of fractures in old age. He did not hazard a guess about the size of the difference, although it might be possible to develop an estimate from the data in Matkovic's study.

Calcium supplementation has several potential effects besides its effects on the skeleton, some beneficial and some harmful. On the beneficial side, evidence is accumulating to show that calcium may help prevent hypertension[20] and colon cancer in some people.[21] On the other side, there are concerns that excessive calcium may increase the frequency of kidney

---

1977; Horsman, Gallagher, Simpson, and Nordin 1977; Nordin, Horsman, Crilly, and others 1980; and Nilas, Christiansen, and Rødbro 1984.

16. Newcomer, Hodgson, McGill, and others 1978; and Pacifici, Droke, and Avioli 1985.

17. Barkin, Wilson, Manuel, and others 1985.

18. Wasnich, Benfante, Yano, and others 1983; Sakhaee, Nicar, Glass, and others 1984; and Transbøl, Christensen, Jensen, and others 1982.

19. Gallagher, Aaron, Horsman, and others 1973; Jowsey and Gershon-Cohen 1964; and Shah, Krishnarao, and Draper 1967.

20. McCarron and Morris 1985; Belizan, Villar, Pineda, and others 1983; Johnson, Smith, and Freudenheim 1985; and Reed, McGee, Yano, and others 1985.

21. Teppo and Saxén 1979; Phillips 1975; Garland, Shekelle, Barret-Connor, and others 1985; Garland and Garland 1980; and Lipkin and Newmark 1985.

stones, impair the body's ability to repair microfractures, lead to calcification of other parts of the body—particularly the arteries, and interfere with the body's use of other nutrients.[22] How often these side effects occur has not been established, and, in some cases, the fragmentary evidence suggests that there may be few serious effects, but, without more definitive studies, they limit enthusiasm for advocating lifelong increases in calcium. The participants suggested there might be other adverse effects—for example, drinking more milk may make people overweight.

Richard S. Rivlin noted that many questions remain unanswered about calcium supplements and how to take them. There are a wide array of supplements and, so far, not enough work has been done to know which the body can use best, as revealed by rates of absorption, storage, excretion, and the like. Nor is it clear what time of day is best to take calcium or whether it should be taken with meals.

It is already known that certain other nutrients, such as fat and salt, and some widely used drugs, interfere with the body's absorption and excretion of calcium. Thus, as several discussants emphasized, calcium is best thought of as part of an optimal diet, rather than as an isolated intervention. In the same vein, Rivlin suggested that some of the possible risks of higher levels of calcium could be offset by other changes in the diet.[23] He also noted that the doses of calcium currently recommended to help prevent hypertension and colon cancer are similar to those for osteoporosis.

Cost-Effectiveness Analysis

Gerry Oster suggested that, in view of the uncertainties about the size of calcium's effect, cost-effectiveness analysis might best be used to show the consequences of the estimates considered most likely on the basis of current research. For example, if lifelong supplementation to bring people to the Recommended Dietary Allowance or higher might reduce fractures by as little as 10 percent, or as much as 50 percent, cost-effectiveness analyses could show the implications of the two extremes. He shared Peck's concern that so much of the literature has examined intermediate outcomes rather than fractures.

22. Nordin 1960; Lutwak and Whedon 1963; Heaney, Saville, and Recker 1975; Knapp 1947; Robertson, Peacock, and Hodgkinson 1979; Dent, Engelbrecht, and Godfrey 1968; Bernstein, Sadowsky, Hegsted, and others 1966; and Snedeker, Smith, and Greger 1982.
23. Rivlin, in press.

He noted that the medical and epidemiological evidence suggests evaluating three possible times for intervention: at the time of bone mass accumulation, during the period of the menopause, and during old age. The evidence points to the first as the most effective, but it could also be the most expensive since it requires supplementation, whether through diet or special supplements, for many decades.

The ultimate outcome of concern in both the medical literature and cost-effectiveness analyses is, of course, fractures. Using Peck's figure that there are approximately 15 million to 20 million people with osteoporosis in the United States, Oster estimated the costs of fractures and the amount that might be saved by intervention. During the 1970s, osteoporosis and vertebral fractures accounted for 1.1 million hospital days and 500,000 doctors' visits every year, for a cost of $14 per person per year with osteoporosis. If the rate of fractures was cut in half by supplementation, $7 per osteoporotic person-year would be saved. Similar calculations for hip fractures suggested savings of $150 per osteoporotic person-year.[24]

In a complete analysis these savings would be combined with the cost of supplementation to arrive at the net cost of intervention. Intervention would have to be applied either to the entire population or to the population particularly at risk for osteoporosis, either of which is larger than the number who ultimately get osteoporosis. Peck indicated that drinking more milk was probably a more expensive way to get calcium than taking supplements; at current Midwest prices it would cost $6 a month per person to provide the same amount of calcium as 500 milligrams of calcium carbonate, which could cost as little as $4 a month.

Oster emphasized that to evaluate the impact of calcium supplementation on capacity to work, it would be necessary to know more about the effects of fractures, especially hip and vertebral fractures, on people's ability to function. This is particularly important to know for the younger group of sufferers, who might be able to work if their disability were not too great.

24. These calculations assume costs of $250 for a day in the hospital and $30 for a doctor's visit.

chapter seven **Alcohol Use**

The use and misuse of alcohol takes many forms, from social drinking to occasional binges to habitual, excessive drinking. In many cases, whether drinking is harmful or not depends on the circumstances in which it takes place—a drink at home may be safe, while one before driving may not be. The discussion at the workshop ranged across the different types of drinking and the very different types of interventions appropriate to them. The participants disagreed over the adequacy and interpretation of the data concerning alcohol use and alcoholism; as a result, they differed in their recommendations about the readiness of the area for cost-effectiveness evaluation.

Health Effects

Most Americans drink alcohol.[1] Gallup polls taken over four decades have consistently reported that about two-thirds of women and three-fourths of men drink at least occasionally. A minority are heavy drinkers— some studies suggest that 10 percent of drinkers account for more than half of the alcohol consumed—and alcoholics are in this minority. Alcoholics represent an important problem for work capacity; their ability to work is seriously and routinely impaired, by their heavy drinking at first, and later by both the drinking and the related health problems.

Donald W. Goodwin noted that excessive drinkers can be defined as those who drink eight or more drinks (four ounces of ethanol) a day.[2] Alcoholics are defined as excessive drinkers who have problems because of their drinking, such as delirium tremens, cirrhosis of the liver, or a

Donald W. Goodwin wrote and presented the background paper. *Ernestine Vanderveen* and *Harold D. Holder* discussed it.
1. Klerman 1982.
2. The definition was proposed by Vaillant 1983.

crime committed under the influence of alcohol. Statistics about alcoholism are suspect, in part because many alcoholics are not truthful
about their drinking, but the best information indicates that 10 million to
15 million Americans are alcoholics, and that perhaps another 35 million suffer indirectly, for example, children in families with an alcoholic
parent.[3]

Goodwin described the consequences of alcoholism as staggering. The
life expectancy of alcoholics is ten to twelve years shorter than the average.[4] A third or more of hospital admissions for men are admissions of
alcoholics, although the hospitalization is usually for reasons other than
alcoholism.[5] While the health effects are major, it can be difficult to link
specific conditions to alcohol because heavy drinkers differ from other
people in many ways. They smoke more, often eat less, and tend not to
exercise or sleep regular hours.

Nonetheless, certain illnesses have been traced to alcohol.[6] The best
known is cirrhosis of the liver, which is the eighth leading cause of death
in the United States. Ten percent to 20 percent of alcoholics develop either
acute hepatitis (inflammation of the liver), which can be fatal, or cirrhosis.
Inflammation of the stomach, called gastritis, is extremely common in
alcoholics. Alcoholics frequently suffer from pain and tingling in the legs,
sometimes accompanied by muscle weakness, and, eventually, by muscle
wasting and paralysis; deficiencies of the B vitamins cause this condition.
Irregular heartbeat, high blood pressure, and malfunction of the heart
ventricles are associated with alcoholism. X-rays of alcoholics' brains
show evidence of atrophy, but since alcoholics have normal IQs and think
clearly when they are sober, the interpretation of this evidence is not yet
clear. A small number of alcoholics suffer definite brain damage because
of a deficiency of thiamine, one of the B vitamins.

Those at greatest risk for becoming alcoholics are people from families
with a history of alcoholism.[7] It was once thought that this connection was
the result of example, but the evidence now suggests a genetic component—people who become alcoholics apparently inherit a susceptibility to
alcohol. Men, and people who were hyperactive as children, are also at
somewhat greater risk of becoming alcoholics.

    3. Brandsma 1980.
    4. Alibrandi 1978; Medhus 1975; and U.S. Public Health Service 1979.
    5. Graham 1982.
    6. Goodwin 1981.
    7. Vaillant 1983

Excessive drinking, either occasional or habitual, has serious health effects that extend beyond the drinkers themselves. It is a major cause of accidents. Alcohol may be involved in almost half of all automobile fatalities, thus helping to cause about 10,000 deaths a year.[8] It is a factor in many motorcycle accidents and in as many as half of all recreational boating deaths.[9] Studies show that 40 percent of adults killed in pedestrian accidents were intoxicated at the time.[10] Alcohol may be involved in half of all homicides and one quarter of suicides.[11] Not only does drinking cause accidents, but there is evidence that the extent of injury from a given accident is greater when the injured person has been drinking.[12]

Moderate drinking can have adverse side effects for the drinker. For example, many Asians suffer low blood pressure, nausea, and facial flush after even a small amount of alcohol. Alcohol itself is high in calories, but has little nutritional value beyond that. Some studies have reported that moderate drinking is associated with small errors in thought and judgment.

The use of alcohol, especially in moderation, has some beneficial effects as well. Over the centuries, it has come to play an important role in cultural and social events, helping to mark rites of passage. It eases everyday tensions for many people, at home and in social gatherings. Some evidence suggests that moderate drinkers have less heart disease and live longer than either heavy drinkers or nondrinkers, although experts disagree over the strength and interpretation of the evidence.

Interventions

Goodwin observed that drastic restrictions on alcohol have succeeded in reducing its use and adverse health effects. During Prohibition the death rate from cirrhosis of the liver declined markedly in the United States. Similarly, alcohol-related health problems declined in Britain and France when alcohol was rationed during World War II. But severe restrictions are hard to maintain, both because of the cultural acceptance of alcohol and because alcohol is easy to make at home. Prohibition was repealed and the wartime restrictions were lifted.

8. Manisses Communications Group 1986, p. 7.
9. Luna, Maier, Sowder, and others 1984; Burnett 1986; and U.S. National Transportation Safety Board 1983.
10. Fell and Hazzard 1985.
11. U.S. Public Health Service 1984, pp. 87 and 93.
12. Waller, Hansen, Stutts, and Popkin 1986.

To prevent the consequences of habitual heavy drinking, the emphasis has turned to treatment of alcoholism once it develops. A wide variety of treatments can be offered singly or in combination. The possibilities include inpatient treatment—with either fixed or variable lengths of stay, outpatient treatment of all kinds, group therapy of all kinds, the use of tranquilizers and Antabuse,[13] halfway houses, drugs that cause nausea when alcohol is consumed, and self-help groups, notably Alcoholics Anonymous.

Hundreds of studies have been conducted over many years testing the effectiveness of various forms of treatment.[14] Goodwin stated that, to date, no form of treatment has been rigorously shown to be superior to any other, or superior to no treatment at all. The most important predictors of whether an alcoholic will be cured are the individual's characteristics— people with stable jobs and marriages, and in the higher socioeconomic classes, do better.

Many of the studies suffer from methodological defects. Virtually none of them includes a control group that did not receive treatment, and few have randomly assigned patients to treatment or control. The patients who receive treatment are generally volunteers. They have decided to try to cure their drinking problem and the decision to enter treatment is a sign of their determination. This determination may well be the critical factor in any cure. Many alcoholics cure themselves without professional help: the spontaneous cure rate may be as high as 25 or 50 percent. Based on the longest and most comprehensive study of a community sample ever conducted, George Vaillant concluded that "alcoholics recover not because we treat them but because they heal themselves."[15]

Despite the consistency of the research results, most investigators, and Goodwin with them, believe that it is worthwhile to continue to treat alcoholism. It is clearly beneficial to cure alcoholism. This is confirmed by studies of the health of recovered alcoholics[16] and by studies showing that the use of medical services by alcoholics declines after they quit drinking.[17] Further, future studies may be able to sort out the factors

13. Antabuse is a drug that makes people ill when they drink.
14. For reviews, see Voegtlin and Lemere 1942; Hill and Blane 1967; Emrick 1974; Emrick 1982; Baekeland, Lundwall, and Kissin 1975; Costello 1982; McCrady and Shear 1983; and Saxe, Dougherty, Esty, and Fine 1983.
15. Vaillant 1983, p. 314.
16. U.S. Public Health Service 1984, p. xvii.
17. Holder 1987.

involved and show that treatment works, or at least some kinds of treatment, for some people.

In her discussion, Ernestine Vanderveen emphasized that some of the misuse of alcohol is not due to habitual heavy drinking but to drinking in inappropriate situations. A large part of the problem of drunk driving could be described as inappropriate use—drinking before driving. Similarly, drinking on the job is often inappropriate—a 1982 study in Maryland found that 11 percent of those killed in job-related accidents were intoxicated.[18] This kind of misuse calls for a different kind of intervention.

Several broad forms of intervention have been aimed at all use of alcohol, both habitual and more occasional. Harold D. Holder discussed the evidence for the effectiveness of two of these—establishing a minimum age for the legal purchase of alcohol, and using taxes to raise the retail price. Restricting advertising and limiting the hours that bars and liquor stores are open are two interventions, not discussed at the workshop, which have also been used.

During the 1970s many states lowered their minimum drinking age to 18. Holder reviewed studies that investigated the effects of the change on traffic deaths.[19] One study, for example, found higher rates of death in traffic accidents in Michigan, Wisconsin, and the province of Ontario, which lowered the purchase age, than in Indiana, Illinois, and Minnesota, which did not.[20] He concluded that a number of studies indicate that an older purchase age reduces deaths and injuries associated with alcohol misuse among youthful drivers.

Some studies also suggest that higher retail prices reduce the consumption of alcohol and its adverse effects.[21] These studies have found lower death rates from cirrhosis and lower rates of traffic deaths where retail prices are higher. The results suggest that higher prices may affect heavy drinkers, not just light or moderate drinkers as some observers expected.

18. U.S. Public Health Service 1984, pp. 131–33.
19. Douglas and Freedman 1977; Williams, Zador, Harris, and Karpf 1983; Cucchiaro, Ferreira, Jr., and Sicherman 1974; Lynn 1981; Cook and Tauchen 1982; Voas and Moulden 1980; Klein 1981; Filkens and Flora 1981; Wagenaar 1983; Wagenaar, forthcoming; U.S. National Highway Traffic Safety Administration 1982; Fell 1983; Williams, Zador, Harris, and Karpf 1981; Hingson, Scotch, Mangione, and others 1983; Smith, Hingson, Morelock, and others 1984; and Lillis, Williams, and Williford, forthcoming.
20. Williams, Zador, Harris, and Karpf 1983.
21. Ornstein and Hanssens 1981; Cook and Tauchen 1982; Levy and Sheflin 1981; Hoadley, Fuchs, and Holder 1984; Cook 1981; Grossman, Coate, and Arluck, forthcoming; and Grossman 1985.

Vanderveen's distinction between habitual misuse and inappropriate use of alcohol suggests the possibility of more specific kinds of intervention— interventions designed to improve safety and performance on the job, at home, or during leisure activities. She noted that heavy drinking could have particularly serious consequences for the performance of tasks requiring a high degree of skill, coordination, and alertness, and gave auto assembly, the operation of construction equipment, and quality-control inspections of nuclear plants as examples. The discussants suggested others—sailing, running a power saw, or climbing a ladder. In some cases it may be possible to design the equipment to help improve safety, but education and social pressure to discourage people from drinking in such situations are also likely to be important. Vanderveen mentioned that school programs, modeled after successful programs to prevent smoking, are being tested on fifth and sixth graders to help them learn to recognize and resist the misuse of alcohol.

Cost-Effectiveness Analysis

Participants in this session disagreed over whether full-scale cost-effectiveness analysis, with changes in work capacity as its focus, is worthwhile in the area of alcohol use at this time. The disagreement centered on whether current studies of alcoholism treatment were adequate to support an evaluation. Goodwin argued that treatment of alcoholism has not yet been proven effective by studies that meet the highest standards for scientific research and thus fails the crucial test for an analysis. Holder and Vanderveen countered that the available studies, while imperfect, show that treatment works for some people.

Evaluations of changes in minimum purchase age and in retail price may be more promising interventions for evaluation. Holder argued that the evidence shows both are effective in reducing the use of alcohol and its consequences. But Goodwin thought that, here again, the studies were not sufficiently rigorous nor consistent in their results to support such a conclusion.

chapter eight   **Obesity**

Obesity is an excess of body fat, not simply, as most laypeople think of it, an excess of weight. While it has been known for years that obesity is associated with poor health, recent research has introduced important refinements of that generalization. It now appears that not only the amount of body fat but its distribution matters; and that the optimal weight is not the same for all ages but increases with age. The discussion at the workshop session suggested that it may be too soon to attempt a general cost-effectiveness analysis of interventions to reduce obesity. Two more specific possibilities were suggested for analysis—surgery for extremely obese people, and appetite depressants as an alternative for obese people who would otherwise have to take antidiabetic or antihypertensive medication.

Health Effects

George A. Bray noted that a wide variety of techniques can be used to measure obesity. The most accurate ones are expensive and impractical for studying large populations or for everyday use. Methods based on height, weight, body measurements, and skinfold measurements—which only approximate obesity—are used for these purposes. The most commonly used are "relative weight" and the "body mass index." Relative weight is an individual's weight expressed as a percentage of the desirable weight for that age, sex, and height; tables of desirable weights allow people to calculate their own relative weights.[1] The body mass index is the individ-

George A. Bray wrote and presented the background paper. *Albert J. Stunkard* and *Brian T. Yates* discussed it.

1. The most widely used tables are those provided by the Metropolitan Life Insurance Company (1959). Bray also recommended the Fogarty table of desirable weights in Bray 1976, p. 7.

ual's weight divided by the square of his or her height; weight is measured in kilograms and height in meters for this index. For example, a woman who is 131 pounds and five feet, seven inches tall has a body mass index of 20.6.[2]

Most studies of the health effects of obesity have used either the relative weight or the body mass index, with the body mass index the more popular of the two. Recent evidence indicates, however, that the distribution of fat may be as important as the total amount in predicting health outcomes. In particular, studies of heart disease show that fat on the trunk is hazardous to health while fat on the hips and thighs is not, at least for this condition.[3] These studies have used the ratio of the circumference of the waist to the circumference of the hips to represent the distribution of fat. Bray recommended that this measurement be included in all future studies of obesity.

Studies of death rates, total and for specific diseases, show that the lowest rates occur for values of the body mass index in the range 20 to 25, approximately the normal weight range. Above this range, and in some cases below it as well, the risk of death is higher. Weights represented by indexes of 25 to 30 extend from the highest weights considered appropriate for people with large frames to about 30 percent overweight. An index of 40 marks the beginning of extreme overweight, which is alternatively defined as 100 percent, or 100 pounds, overweight.

Studies based on data collected by life insurance companies were the first to show that overweight is associated with higher death rates.[4] Over the last several decades a number of large, prospective studies, in which initially healthy populations are followed for a number of years, have confirmed the relationship and shown that overweight precedes disease and thus is the cause of it.[5] The study of the population of Framingham, Massachusetts, which has been central to so many health debates, the American Cancer Society study, and several studies done in Scandinavia show that death rates are lowest for people whose body mass index is in

2. A kilogram is 2.20 pounds and a meter is 39.37 inches. Her weight in kilograms is thus 59.5, her height in meters is 1.70, and her height squared is 2.89 meters, for a ratio of weight to height squared of 20.6.

3. Lapidus, Bengtsson, Larsson, and others 1984; and Kissebah, Vydelingum, Murray and others 1982.

4. Bray 1982; and Society of Actuaries 1979.

5. The Pooling Project Research Group 1978; Hubert, Feinleib, McNamara, and Castelli 1983; Feinleib 1985; Kannel and Gordon 1979; Lew and Garfinkel 1979; Larsson, Björntorp, and Tibblin 1981; Lapidus, Bengtsson, Larsson, and others 1984; and Waaler 1983.

the range 20 to 25 or 27, and the rise is approximately linear for higher weights. The risk associated with obesity is greater for men and for younger people.[6]

One of the difficulties in interpreting these data is that, apparently, less attention has been given than in other areas of prevention to estimating the independent effect of obesity, that is, its effect over and above that of other unhealthy characteristics of the individual. The American Cancer Society study does show, however, that the effects of smoking are considerably more severe than those of obesity. A nonsmoker would have to have a body mass index of 35, which represents 60 to 70 excess pounds, to have the same risk of death as a smoker of normal weight. Another problem in interpreting the data is that it has only recently been accepted that the optimal weight is not the same for all ages, but is higher for older people.[7] This may be part of the reason that the risks of overweight are greater for younger people than for those who put on weight later in life.

The strongest link is between obesity and diabetes. The American Cancer Society data show that death rates from diabetes are lowest at a body mass index of 24 to 26 and that they are eight times that rate at an index of 35.[8] Gallbladder disease shows the next strongest association, with the risk of death for overweight people two to four times that of normal-weight people, depending on the study; underweight people are also at higher risk for gallbladder disease. The risks of death from cardiovascular disease and cancer also rise with weight, but not so steeply. For example, the highest risk with cancer is only 1.2 times to 1.5 times the lowest risk; higher risks show up for breast, cervical, ovarian, and gallbladder cancers in women, and for colorectal and prostatic cancers in men. For a while, it was thought that obesity might not be an independent factor in cardiovascular disease, but a recent analysis of the Framingham experience shows that it is.[9]

The effect of obesity on illness and disability, which are of particular importance for people's ability to work, does not appear to have been studied in as much detail as its effects on death rates. It is generally

6. Abraham, Collins, and Nordsieck 1971; and Drenick, Bale, Seltzer, and Johnson, 1980.

7. Andres, Elahi, Tobin, and others 1985.

8. Lew and Garfinkel 1979. The relative weights reported in the article were translated into values of the body mass index on the basis of calculations by Lew.

9. Hubert, Feinlieb, McNamara, and Castelli 1983.

accepted that obesity contributes to hypertension.[10] And a Scandinavian study concluded that "even moderate obesity increases the risk for hypertension, diabetes mellitus, gallstone disease, kidney-stone disease, and cerebrovascular disease," conditions that cause disability as well as premature death. The same study found no connection between obesity and either angina or peptic ulcer.[11]

Interventions

Obesity, measured approximately by overweight, is a very prevalent condition in the United States. A consensus conference convened by the National Institutes of Health agreed that being 20 percent overweight was a health hazard, and that a lower degree of overweight could be a problem if it occurred together with disease.[12] Data collected in the United States in the late 1960s and 1970s show that about one quarter of all adults were overweight by roughly 20 percent or more.[13] Older people were more likely to be overweight than younger people—the percentage rose from about 10 percent for those in their early 20s to more than one quarter for middle-aged or older men and more than one-third for women 55 or older. People of low socioeconomic status are more likely to be overweight, and so are people from certain cultural backgrounds, particularly those from Eastern Europe.[14] Obesity has recently started to increase among children, and this is likely to be reflected in more obesity among adults in the future.[15]

A wide range of interventions is available to combat overweight. For extreme cases, surgery to restrict the capacity of the stomach is successful. Appetite depressants have long been considered useful for short-term weight loss and may turn out to be appropriate for long-term use in some people. There is a bewildering array of diets, which can be combined with varying amounts and types of exercise and various behavioral techniques to help the dieter stay with it.

10. Bray 1982; and U.S. Department of Health, Education, and Welfare 1979.
11. Larsson, Björntorp, and Tibblin 1981.
12. U.S. National Institutes of Health 1985.
13. U.S. National Center for Health Statistics 1983; and unpublished data from the second National Health and Nutrition Examination Survey, 1976–80, U.S. National Center for Health Statistics, Division of Health Examination Statistics.
14. Goldblatt, Moore, and Stunkard 1965.
15. U.S. National Institutes of Health 1985.

Bray reviewed some of the evidence that weight loss leads to better health, but described it as "not very impressive." Life insurance data show that people who were overweight when they applied for a first policy, but who had fallen to normal weight before applying a second time, had the life expectancies of normal-weight people.[16] One prospective study measured glucose tolerance in a group of people over ten years; those who remained normal or improved their glucose tolerance were also those who maintained or lowered their weight.[17] An analysis of data from Framingham showed that cholesterol, glucose, uric acid, and blood pressure all rose in those who gained weight and declined in those who lost it.[18] Other studies have also shown that a reduction in blood pressure usually follows weight loss.[19] During periods of rationing and deprivation in World War II, hypertension was almost nonexistent.

Albert J. Stunkard described several programs he has tested for encouraging large numbers of people to lose weight. The most successful to date is a "weight-loss competition," in which the employees of different companies compete against each other to see who can lose the most pounds. Those employees who qualify to participate (by being overweight) are given an individual weight-loss goal, and the team effort reflects the success of each employee. Stunkard's group has developed a manual that allows businesses to mount their own competitions with a minimum of help from outside experts.

A problem with weight loss programs, as with smoking cessation programs, is that people succeed for a time and then fall back into their old habits. A few recent studies have followed people for long enough after the initial weight loss to indicate what the longer-term success rate can be. On the basis of five to fourteen years of follow-up, they indicate that as many as 25 percent to 35 percent of those who lose weight keep it off.[20]

Bray described one hypothesis for overweight that points to a particular kind of diet for maintaining proper weight. The nutrient imbalance hypothesis starts with the premise that the body regulates particular nutrients rather than total caloric intake. The intake of carbohydrates and protein is regulated very closely, and the body tries to maintain the proper balance

16. Society of Actuaries 1979. See also Hubert, Feinlieb, McNamara, and Castelli 1983; Feinleib 1985; and Kannel and Gordon 1979.

17. Toeller, Gries, and Dannehl 1982.

18. Ashley and Kannel 1974.

19. Dustan 1985; Reisin, Abel, Modan, and others 1978; and Tuck, Sowers, Dornfeld, and others 1981.

20. Stunkard and Penick 1979; and Sohar and Sneh 1973.

from day to day. The intake of fat is regulated over much longer periods of time and much less closely. This pattern suggests that a diet high in carbohydrates and low in fat should make it more difficult to become overweight.[21]

Cost-Effectiveness Analysis

Stunkard thought the time was not right for a general cost-effectiveness analysis of losing weight. The heterogeneity of the disorder, the variety of treatments, and the problem of recidivism all pose obstacles to an analysis. He thought the health effects of proper weight would be clearer when more work has been done taking into account the newly discovered importance of the distribution of fat and the desirability of an increase in weight with age.

In the meantime, he suggested that two specific groups were ready for analysis. The first group is the extremely obese (also called the morbidly obese)—people who are 100 percent or one hundred pounds overweight. This group is very small, about 0.5 percent of all obese people, and 0.2 percent of the total population. Good results have been obtained with surgery for this group; vertical banded gastroplasty is the best of the available surgical techniques.[22] Good data are available on the illness and disability suffered by the extremely obese, on the costs and risks of surgery, and on the improvement in ability to function following surgery. The improvements are often dramatic—people who were virtually unable to function before are able to return to work or to their former activities.[23]

The second possibility for analysis is the use of appetite depressants as a substitute for antidiabetic or antihypertensive medication. It used to be thought that people developed a tolerance for appetite depressants that made them ineffective for long-term use, but recent work has shown this is not true.[24] For most people, long-term use would still be considered undesirable on the ground that it involves unknown but potentially serious risks. But many people are already committed to taking medication to

21. Bray 1987.
22. Vertical banded gastroplasty is a surgical procedure designed to restrict the capacity of the stomach (to as little as half an ounce) in an effort to decrease meal size and total food intake.
23. Stunkard, Stinnett, and Smoller 1986; and Stunkard, Foster, and Grossman 1986.
24. Stunkard 1982.

control their hypertension or diabetes. Since weight loss is often enough to control diabetes or lower blood pressure, appetite depressants offer an alternative way to achieve the same results. A multicenter trial is under way in Europe to test the health effects of this alternative, and a cost-effectiveness analysis could evaluate the effects relative to the costs.[25]

Brian T. Yates suggested several general strategies for evaluating the cost-effectiveness of interventions to control obesity and for improving the cost-effectiveness of their application. He indicated that research needed to focus on which of the many possible elements of a weight reduction program—group meetings, exercise, counseling, diet advice, and so on—do the most to reduce weight.[26] Available treatments could be ranked in order of their cost-effectiveness, and the most cost-effective could be tried first; for people who did not respond, further treatments could be tried, proceeding up the scale to more expensive alternatives. It may also eventually be possible to assign people to treatments on the basis of their previous history of failures or according to the particular genetic and environmental risks they face.

Yates also noted the importance of looking at cost-effectiveness from the perspective of the individual as well as society. The costs faced by the individual—these include inconvenience and discomfort—are an important factor in his or her decision to stay with the intervention.

The session ended with a discussion of the pitfalls of focusing on intermediate outcomes—pounds of weight lost, points of reduction in blood pressure, and the like. David Siscovick noted that it is often easier to study intermediate outcomes because they change more quickly than the ultimate outcomes of disease and death. Gerry Oster warned, however, that concentrating on intermediate outcomes runs the risk that they will be viewed as the goal. In order not to lose sight of the true goal—better health and longer life—studies should try to estimate health effects in those terms.

25. Albert J. Stunkard, personal communication.
26. Yates 1978, and forthcoming.

appendix   **Guidelines for Cost-Effectiveness**
               Evaluations

          The purpose of an evaluation is to help policymakers
decide whether a particular strategy represents a good investment of time
and money. Implicitly or explicitly, the benefits of the strategy are compared with the benefits of other ways of using the same resources. Comparisons are thus crucial to the decision. To facilitate these comparisons,
cost-effectiveness evaluations of major preventive strategies should be
based as much as possible on the same principles and basic assumptions.
          This appendix recommends a common core of principles and assump-
tions to guide future evaluations, including those that may be undertaken
as a result of the workshop.

What Cost-Effectiveness Analysis Is

Cost-effectiveness analysis is a set of methods for measuring and comparing the costs and health effects of a specified change. When a medical
intervention is evaluated, the outlays for the intervention are calculated,
and any savings because medical care or other costs are avoided as a result
of the intervention are subtracted. The health effects of the intervention
have traditionally been measured in lives saved, years of life saved, or
cases of disease avoided. In more recent studies, health effects are sometimes summarized in terms of well-years, a measure that allows for
changes in pain and suffering, and in illness and disability, as well as in
length of life (see the discussion of well-years in chapter 3). Any losses of
life or health because of side effects of the intervention are subtracted from
the gains to arrive at net health effects.

Louise B. Russell developed these guidelines. They were not discussed at the workshop
for lack of time, but they were circulated to all the participants.

The costs and health effects of the intervention can be summarized more formally. Costs equal

—the costs of the intervention

—plus the costs of treating its side effects

—minus savings in future medical costs because disease is prevented.

Health effects equal

—the years of life added by the intervention

—plus improvements in health during years that would have been lived anyway, because nonfatal disease is also prevented by the intervention;

—minus any deterioration in health because of side effects of the intervention.

The cost-effectiveness ratio is then defined as costs divided by health effects:

$$\text{cost-effectiveness ratio} = \frac{\text{costs}}{\text{health effects}}$$
$$= \text{cost per unit of health effect}$$

Depending on the way health gains are measured, the cost-effectiveness ratio could be the cost per life saved, per year of life, per case of disease prevented, or per well-year.

Besides the cost-effectiveness ratio, the results of a cost-effectiveness evaluation are generally presented in detailed tables showing costs and effects by type of cost, by age or risk of the people affected, and so on.[1] The tables give a sense for what actually underlies the ratios—who benefits and how and what sorts of costs are incurred.

Guidelines

The recommended guidelines can be grouped under three headings: the framework of the study, health effects, and costs.[2]

The Framework of the Study

To set the framework of the study, the analyst must choose an appropriate perspective, a discount rate, and a way of indicating the imprecision of the estimates.

1. For example, see Berwick and Komaroff 1982; or Weinstein and Stason 1976.
2. For a fuller discussion of many of these recommendations, see Russell 1986.

PERSPECTIVE OF THE STUDY.   The logical perspective for public policy is that of society as a whole, rather than some segment of society such as employers, insurers, federal programs, or even individuals. The difference between these partial perspectives and that of society is that the social perspective counts all gains in health, net of any losses, regardless of who enjoys the gains or suffers the losses. And it counts all costs, net of savings, regardless of who incurs the costs or pockets the savings.

DISCOUNT RATE.   The discount rate can have a major effect on the results of a cost-effectiveness study, and it is impossible to make valid comparisons among studies that use different discount rates.[3] Thus all studies should use the same discount rate or rates. And since all the dollar amounts in a cost-effectiveness analysis are in real terms, that is, net of inflation, the discount rate must also be in real terms.

Most studies in the literature use 4, 5, or 6 percent. While the discount rate represents an important value judgment—a judgment about the desirability of future benefits and costs compared with present ones—the rates actually used seem to be a matter of convention. They are too close to signal any real disagreement on the appropriate rate. Cost-effectiveness evaluations should show results for two rates—5 percent and zero. Zero is the extreme case of no discounting; it shows how much the results can change as the discount rate is reduced and suggests whether the value judgment implicit in the rate chosen is important for the results of the particular study.

IMPRECISION OF THE ESTIMATES.   The estimates produced by a cost-effectiveness study are not exact. Instead they represent a range of possible values. Some notion of the size of that range is desirable.

Most studies do sensitivity analyses, that is, they present estimates for values of important variables—such as the incidence of the condition, or the gain from prevention—other than those used in the base case. It can be particularly illuminating to do sensitivity analyses for groups of assumptions that are more pessimistic or optimistic than the base case. For example, the pessimistic case might include an assumption that the effectiveness of prevention is one standard deviation lower than the most likely value, and that certain important costs are one standard deviation higher than their most likely values. It is preferable to choose values that are, say, one standard deviation from the most likely value because these values

3. Cretin (1977) demonstrated that the effect of discounting can be particularly important for prevention, since it often does not produce benefits until many years after the costs have been incurred.

have a reasonably high probability of being true. The extreme values of the range, such as the lowest possible value for effectiveness, give an unduly pessimistic picture of the uncertainty of the estimates since they are, in fact, very unlikely to be true.

Health Effects

MODELING HEALTH EFFECTS. The effectiveness of a change in health habits is fundamentally important because the change must be effective before it can be cost-effective. That is, it must have some beneficial effects on health before there is any point to considering its costs, either alone or in relation to the health effects.

A cost-effectiveness study cannot estimate either health effects or costs well unless patterns of the incidence of disease, the outcomes of disease, and the good and bad effects of change/intervention are modeled well. Thus it is of the first importance to do a good job of modeling effectiveness, using the best available information about health effects. The purpose of the workshop was precisely to identify the best available information and determine whether it is good enough to warrant cost-effectiveness evaluations.

MEASURING QUALITY AS WELL AS QUANTITY OF HEALTH. If studies are to be comparable, they must use the same measure of effects, and to accommodate all studies (as well as the way people actually judge health), that measure must allow for changes in the quality as well as the quantity of life. The well-year, described in chapter 3, and its variants offer a practical way to accommodate these needs.

To reap the full benefit of the method, consistent sets of weights need to be used in different studies so that, for example, side effects from antihypertensive medication are not overweighted (or underweighted) relative to the quality of life with angina. The results of sample surveys have shown that such weights can be developed.[4] These surveys can serve as a direct source of weights for some studies and as a benchmark for the weights needed for studies of conditions that may not be well represented in them.

FUTURE EARNINGS. It is often of interest to know the future earnings that may result because changes in health habits make people healthier and able to work longer. Earnings must, however, be handled carefully in a

4. Kaplan, Bush, and Berry 1978.

cost-effectiveness study, and it is important to be clear about their place in the study and their proper interpretation.

Estimates of earnings should not be deducted from the costs of an intervention. Earnings are only one of the ways that gains in health can be used. The additional time and energy can also be used to go to school, care for children or older relatives, do volunteer work, engage in recreational activities, and so on. All these gains, or, rather, the raw material with which they would be produced, are already counted in the form of well-years or in the cruder form of lives or years of life saved. To include earnings in the cost-effectiveness calculations is to count part of the health effects twice—once as a gain in health and again as a saving subtracted from program costs.

Estimates of future earnings should be viewed instead as providing additional detail about the health gains. Estimates could be made as well of the other ways in which the additional health might be used.

Costs

MEDICAL COSTS IN ADDED YEARS OF LIFE.   Besides the medical costs associated with a preventive measure and any savings because disease is prevented, some studies also include the medical expenses incurred because a person lives longer. This is appropriate if the issue is how prevention will affect total expenditures for medical care, an issue of considerable interest to many people.

But this is a narrow issue, one that does not truly reflect society's perspective. When the question is instead simply whether the proposed strategy is a good use of resources, all resources used directly for the strategy should be counted as costs, whether those resources are used in the medical sector or elsewhere. The strategy's *indirect* effects on medical expenditures are no more relevant than its indirect effects on expenditures for food, clothes, or housing, all of which increase when people live longer. Like future earnings, future medical expenses are one of the indirect consequences of the health gains. Estimates of them might be presented as an elaboration of those consequences, but not as an addition to them or to costs.

In general, the estimates should exclude medical expenditures in added years of life. A second set of estimates including them could be made as well because of the widespread interest in the effect of prevention on total medical expenditures, but these estimates should be clearly identified as relevant only to that narrower issue.

COSTS OUTSIDE THE MEDICAL SECTOR.   Cost-effectiveness studies in health have focused on interventions for which medical costs are the only or the primary costs. For many preventive interventions, however, costs outside of medical care will be important, either as outlays or as savings.

Institutionalization and special education are sometimes included in cost-effectiveness analyses when the intervention under consideration can prevent retardation and other disabilities, thus producing savings. Exercise is a good example of an intervention that requires substantial costs outside medical care.

For costs outside of medical care, as for medical costs, the social perspective dictates that the net costs of a change be measured. For example, the net costs of institutionalization are the costs over and above the costs if the same person lived at home; the rest are matched by savings elsewhere in the economy. Similarly, the relevant costs of special education are the costs over and above those for a normal education. Any savings due to prevention are thus these net amounts, not the full costs of institutionalization or special education. The same principle applies to less familiar types of costs, such as those for exercise. If it were possible to figure out what people would do if they were not exercising—perhaps watch television or go to the movies—the costs of that activity could be subtracted from the costs associated with exercise.

Summary

Cost-effectiveness evaluations of preventive strategies should
—Adopt the social perspective;
—Use a discount rate of 5 percent;
—Perform sensitivity analyses of sets of assumptions that represent cases more optimistic and pessimistic than the base case;
—Give particular attention to modeling health effects carefully;
—Use the well-year to summarize health effects;
—Treat estimates of future earnings as amplification of the possible consequences of the health effects and not as an item to be subtracted from costs;
—Omit medical costs in added years of life; and
—Estimate all costs and savings of a change in health habits, including those that fall outside the medical sector.

Bibliography

How to Model Health Effects

Casale, P. N., R. B. Devereux, M. Milner, and others. "Value of Echocardiographic Measurement of Left Ventricular Mass in Predicting Cardiovascular Morbid Events in Hypertensive Men." *Annals of Internal Medicine,* vol. 105 (1986), pp. 173–78.

Dawber, T. R. *The Framingham Study: The Epidemiology of Atherosclerotic Disease.* Cambridge: Harvard University Press, 1980.

Hypertension Detection and Follow-up Program Cooperative Group. "Five-Year Findings of the Hypertension Detection and Follow-up Program: Reduction in Mortality of Persons with High Blood Pressure, Including Mild Hypertension." *Journal of the American Medical Association,* vol. 242 (1979), pp. 2562–71.

Joint National Committee on Detection, Evaluation, and Treatment of High Blood Pressure. "The 1984 Report of the Joint National Committee on Detection, Evaluation, and Treatment of High Blood Pressure," *Archives of Internal Medicine,* vol. 144 (1984), pp. 1045–57.

MacMahon, S. W., D. E. L. Wilcken, and G. J. Macdonald. "The Effect of Weight Reduction on Left Ventricular Mass. A Randomized Controlled Trial in Young, Overweight Hypertensive Patients." *New England Journal of Medicine,* vol. 314 (1986), pp. 334–39.

Management Committee. "The Australian Therapeutic Trial in Mild Hypertension." *Lancet,* vol. 1 (1980), pp. 1261–67.

Medical Research Council Working Party. "Adverse Reactions to Bendrofluazide and Propranolol for the Treatment of Mild Hypertension." *Lancet* vol. 2 (1981), pp. 539–43.

———. "MRC Trial of Treatment of Mild Hypertension: Principal Results." *British Medical Journal,* vol. 291 (1985), pp. 97–104.

Multiple Risk Factor Intervention Trial Research Group. "Multiple Risk

Factor Intervention Trial: Risk Factor Changes and Mortality Results." *Journal of the American Medical Association,* vol. 248 (1982), pp. 1465-77.

Savage, D. D., R. D. Abbott, S. Padget, and others. "Epidemiologic Features of Left Ventricular Hypertrophy in Normotensive and Hypertensive Subjects." In *Cardiac Left Ventricular Hypertrophy,* edited by H. E. D. J. ter Keurs and J. J. Shipperheyn, pp. 2-15. The Hague: Martinus Nijhoff, 1983.

Savage, D. D., W. P. Castelli, R. D. Abbott, and others. "Hypertrophic Cardiomyopathy and Its Markers in the General Population—the Great Masquerader Revisited: The Framingham Study." *Journal of Cardiovascular Ultrasonography,* vol. 2 (1983), pp. 411-47.

Savage, D. D., J. I. M. Drayer, W. L. Henry, and others. "Echocardiographic Assessment of Cardiac Anatomy and Function in Hypertensive Subjects." *Circulation,* vol. 59 (1979), pp. 623-32.

Savage, D. D., R. J. Garrison, W. P. Castelli, and others. "Echocardiographic Left Ventricular Hypertrophy in the General Population Is Associated with Increased Two-Year Mortality, Independent of Standard Coronary Risk Factors—The Framingham Study." *American Heart Association Council on Cardiovascular Epidemiology Newsletter,* vol. 37 (1985), p. 33.

Topol, E. J., T. A. Traill, and N. J. Fortuin. "Hypertensive Hypertrophic Cardiomyopathy of the Elderly." *New England Journal of Medicine,* vol. 312 (1985), pp. 277-83.

Weinstein, M. C., and W. B. Stason. *Hypertension: A Policy Perspective.* Cambridge: Harvard University Press, 1976.

———. "Economic Considerations in the Management of Mild Hypertension." *Annals of the New York Academy of Sciences,* vol. 304 (1978), pp. 424-40.

World Health Organization. "1986 Guidelines for the Treatment of Mild Hypertension: Memorandum from a WHO/ISH Meeting." *Bulletin of the WHO,* vol. 64 (1986), pp. 31-35.

How to Translate Health Effects

Amberg, J. M., L. J. Schneiderman, C. C. Berry, and others. "The Abnormal Outpatient Chemistry Panel Serum Alkaline Phosphatase: Analysis of Physical Response, Outcome, Cost, and Health Effectiveness." *Journal of Chronic Diseases,* vol. 35 (1982), pp. 81-88.

Anderson, J. P., and R. J. Moser. "Parasite Screening and Treatment Among Indochinese Refugees" *Journal of the American Medical Association*, vol. 253 (1985), pp. 2229–35.

Atkins, C. J., R. M. Kaplan, R. M. Timms, and others. "Behavioral Programs in the Management of Chronic Obstructive Pulmonary Disease." *Journal of Consulting and Clinical Psychology*, vol. 52 (1984), pp. 591–603.

Avery, A. D., T. Lelah, N. E. Solomon, and others. *Quality of Medical Care Assessment Using Outcome Measures: Eight Disease-Specific Applications*. R-2021/2-HEW. Santa Monica, Calif.: Rand Corp., 1976.

Bush, J. W., M. Chen, and D. L. Patrick. "Cost-effectiveness Using a Health Status Index: Analysis of the New York State PKU Screening Program." In *Health Status Indexes*, edited by R. Berg. Chicago: Hospital Research and Educational Trust, 1973.

Chen, M. M., J. W. Bush, and D. L. Patrick. "Social Indicators for Health Planning and Policy Analysis." *Policy Sciences*, vol. 6 (1975), pp. 71–89.

Epstein, K. A., L. D. Schneiderman, J. W. Bush, and others. "The 'Abnormal' Screening Serum Thyroxin (T4): Analysis of Physician Response, Outcome, Cost, and Health Effectiveness." *Journal of Chronic Diseases*, vol. 34 (1981), pp. 175–90.

Fanshel, S., and J. W. Bush. "A Health Status Index and Its Applications to Health-services Outcomes." *Operations Research*, vol. 18 (1970), pp. 1021–66.

Kaplan, R. M. "Human Preference Measurement for Health Decisions and the Evaluation of Long-term Care." In *Values and Long-term Care*, edited by R. L. Kane and R. A. Kane, pp. 157–88. Lexington, Mass.: Lexington Books, 1982.

Kaplan, R. M., C. J. Atkins, and R. M. Timms. "Validity of a Quality of Well-being Scale as an Outcome Measure in Chronic Obstructive Pulmonary Disease." *Journal of Chronic Diseases*, vol. 37 (1984), pp. 85–95.

Kaplan, R. M., and J. W. Bush. "Health-related Quality of Life Measurement for Evaluation Research and Policy Analysis." *Health Psychology*, vol. 1 (1982), pp. 61–80.

Kaplan, R. M., J. W. Bush, and C. C. Berry. "Health Status: Types of Validity for an Index of Well-being." *Health Services Research*, vol. 11 (1976), pp. 478–507.

———. "The Reliability, Stability, and Generalizability of a Health Status

Index." In American Statistical Association, *Proceedings of the Social Statistics Section*, pp. 704–09. Washington, D.C.: American Statistical Association, 1978.

Manton, K. G. "Past and Future Life Expectancy Increases at Later Ages: Their Implications for the Linkage of Chronic Morbidity, Disability and Mortality." *Journal of Gerontology,* vol. 41 (1986), pp. 672–81.

Spiegelman, M. *Introduction to Demography.* Cambridge: Harvard University Press, 1969.

Toevs, C. T., R. M. Kaplan, and C. J. Atkins. "The Costs and Effects of Behavioral Programs in Chronic Obstructive Pulmonary Disease." *Medical Care,* vol 22 (1984), pp. 1088–1100.

Woodbury, M. A., and K. G. Manton. "A Random Walk Model of Human Mortality and Aging." *Theoretical Population Biology,* vol. 11 (1977), pp. 37–48.

Woodbury, M. A., and K. G. Manton. "A New Procedure for Analysis of Medical Classification." *Methods of Information Medicine,* vol. 21 (1982), pp. 210–20.

U.S. Senate. Special Committee on Aging. *The Supplemental Security Income Program: A Ten-Year Overview.* S. Rept. 98-194. 98 Cong. 2 sess. Washington, D.C.: Government Printing Office, 1984.

Smoking

Best, E. W. R., G. H. Josie, and C. B. Walker. "A Canadian Study of Mortality in Relation to Smoking Habits: A Preliminary Report." *Canadian Journal of Public Health,* vol. 52 (1961), pp. 99–106.

Canadian Department of National Health and Welfare. *A Canadian Study of Smoking and Health.* Ottawa: DNHW, 1966.

Cederlof, R., L. Friberg, Z. Hrubec, and V. Lorich. *The Relationship of Smoking and Some Social Covariables to Mortality and Cancer Morbidity. A Ten Year Follow- up in a Probability Sample of 55,000 Swedish Subjects Age 18 to 69. Part I and II.* Stockholm: Karolinska Institute, Department of Environmental Hygiene, 1975.

Doll, R., and A. B. Hill. "Lung Cancer and Other Causes of Death in Relation to Smoking. A Second Report on the Mortality of British Doctors." *British Medical Journal,* vol. 2 (1956), pp. 1071–81.

———. "Mortality in Relation to Smoking: Ten Years' Observations of British Doctors," part 1. *British Medical Journal,* vol. 1 (1964a), pp. 1399–1410.

————. "Mortality in Relation to Smoking: Ten Years' Observations of British Doctors," part 2. *British Medical Journal,* vol. 1 (1964b), pp. 1460–67.

————. "Mortality of British Doctors in Relation to Smoking: Observations on Coronary Thrombosis." In *Epidemiological Approaches to the Study of Cancer and Other Chronic Diseases,* edited by W. Haenszel. National Cancer Institute Monograph 19. Washington, D.C.: U.S. Department of Health, Education, and Welfare, 1966.

Doll, R., and R. Peto. "Mortality in Relation to Smoking: 20 Years' Observations on Male British Doctors." *British Medical Journal,* vol. 2 (1976), pp. 1525–36.

————. "Mortality Among Doctors in Different Occupations." *British Medical Journal,* vol. 2 (1977), pp. 1433–36.

Doll, R., and M. C. Pike. "Trends in Mortality Among British Doctors in Relation to Their Smoking Habits." *Journal of the Royal College of Physicians,* vol. 6 (1972), pp. 216–22.

Dorn, H. F. "The Mortality of Smokers and Nonsmokers." In American Statistical Association, *Proceedings of the Social Statistics Section,* pp. 34–71. Washington, D.C.: American Statistical Association, 1958.

Dunn, J. E., Jr., G. Linden, and L. Breslow. "Lung Cancer Mortality Experience of Men in Certain Occupations in California." *American Journal of Public Health,* vol. 50 (1960), pp. 1475–87.

Hammond, E.C. "Evidence on the Effects of Giving Up Cigarette Smoking." *American Journal of Public Health,* vol. 55 (1965), pp. 682–91.

————. "Smoking in Relation to the Death Rates of One Million Men and Women." In *Epidemiological Approaches to the Study of Cancer and Other Chronic Diseases,* edited by W. Haenszel. National Cancer Institute Monograph 19. Washington, D.C.: HEW, 1966.

————. "Smoking Habits and Air Pollution in Relation to Lung Cancer." In *Environmental Factors in Respiratory Disease,* edited by D. H. K. Lee, pp. 177–98. Fogarty International Center Proceedings No. 11. New York: Academic Press, 1972.

Hammond, E. C., and L. Garfinkel. "Coronary Heart Disease, Stroke, and Aortic Aneurysm: Factors in the Etiology." *Archives of Environmental Health,* vol. 19 (1969), pp. 167–82.

Hammond, E. C., L. Garfinkel, H. Seidman, and others. " 'Tar' and Nicotine Content of Cigarette Smoke in Relation to Death Rates." *Environmental Research,* vol. 12 (1976), pp. 263–74.

Hammond, E. C., and D. Horn. "Smoking and Death Rates—Report on

Forty-four Months of Follow-up of 187,783 Men: Total Mortality." *Journal of the American Medical Association,* vol. 166 (1958), pp. 1159–72.

Hirayama, T. *Smoking in Relation to the Death Rates of 265,118 Men and Women in Japan.* Tokyo: National Cancer Center, 1967.

———. "Smoking and Drinking—Is There a Connection?" *Smoke Signals,* vol. 16 (1970), pp. 1–8.

———. *Smoking in Relation to the Death Rates of 265,118 Men and Women in Japan. A Report on Five Years of Follow-up.* Presented at the American Cancer Society's Fourteenth Science Writers' Seminar, Clearwater Beach, Florida, March 24–29, 1972.

———. "Operational Aspects of Cancer Public Education in Japan." In *Summary Proceedings of the International Conference on Public Education about Cancer,* pp. 85–90. UICC Technical Report Series, vol. 18. Geneva, 1975.

Holbrook, J. H. "Tobacco." In *Harrison's Principles of Internal Medicine,* 11th ed., edited by E. Braunwald and K. J. Isselbacher, pp. 855–59. New York: McGraw-Hill, 1987.

Kahn, H. A. "The Dorn Study of Smoking and Mortality Among U.S. Veterans: Report on Eight and One-half Years of Observation." In *Epidemiological Approaches to the Study of Cancer and Other Chronic Diseases,* edited by W. Haenszel, pp. 1–125. National Cancer Institute Monograph 19. Washington, D.C.: HEW, 1966.

Kuller, L., E. Meilahn, M. Townsend, and others. "Control of Cigarette Smoking from a Medical Perspective." *Annual Review of Public Health,* vol. 3 (1982), pp. 153–78.

Office of Technology Assessment, U.S. Congress. "Staff Memo: Smoking-related Deaths and Financial Costs." Washington, D.C., September 1985.

Rogot, E. *Smoking and General Mortality Among U.S. Veterans, 1954–1969.* DHEW Publication No. (NIH) 75-544. U.S. Department of Health, Education, and Welfare, National Institutes of Health, National Heart and Lung Institute, Epidemiology Branch, 1974a.

Rogot, E. "Smoking and Mortality Among U.S. Veterans," *Journal of Chronic Diseases,* vol. 27 (1974b), pp. 189–203.

U. S. National Center for Health Statistics. *Smoking Data Guide from the National Center for Health Statistics, 1964–84.* Washington, D.C.: Department of Health and Human Services (HHS), 1986.

U. S. Public Health Service. *Smoking and Health: A Report of the Sur-*

geon General. DHEW (PHS) 79-50066. Washington, D.C.: Department of Health, Education, and Welfare (HEW), 1979.

————. *Smoking, Tobacco, and Health: A Fact Book.* DHHS (PHS) 80-50150. Washington, D.C.: HHS, 1981.

————. *The Health Consequences of Smoking: Cancer, A Report of the Surgeon General.* DHHS (PHS) 82-50179. Washington, D.C.: HHS, 1982.

————. *The Health Consequences of Smoking: Cardiovascular Disease, A Report of the Surgeon General, 1983.* DHHS (PHS) 84-50204. Washington, D.C.: HHS, 1984.

————. *The Health Consequences of Smoking: Chronic Obstructive Lung Disease, A Report of the Surgeon General, 1984.* DHHS (PHS) 84-50205. Washington, D.C.: HHS, 1984.

U. S. Surgeon General's Advisory Committee on Smoking and Health. *Smoking and Health: Report of the Advisory Committee to the Surgeon General of the Public Health Service.* PHS 1103. Washington, D.C.: HEW, 1964.

Weir, J. M., and J. E. Dunn, Jr. "Smoking and Mortality: A Prospective Study." *Cancer,* vol. 25 (1970), pp. 105–12.

Winkelstein, W., Jr. "Some Ecological Studies of Lung Cancer and Ischaemic Heart Disease Mortality in the United States." *International Journal of Epidemiology,* vol. 14 (1985), pp. 39–47.

Exercise

Aloia, J. F. "Exercise and Skeletal Health." *Journal of the American Geriatrics Society,* vol. 29 (1981), pp. 104–07.

Aloia, J. F., S. H. Cohn, T. Babu, and others. "Skeletal Mass and Body Composition in Marathon Runners." *Metabolism: Clinical and Experimental,* vol. 27 (1978), pp. 1793–96.

Åstrand, I. "Aerobic Work Capacity in Men and Women with Special Reference to Age." *Acta Physiologica Scandinavica,* vol. 49, supplement 169 (1960), pp. 1–92.

Blair, S. N., N. N. Goodyear, L. W. Gibbons, and K. H. Cooper. "Physical Fitness and Incidence of Hypertension in Healthy Normotensive Men and Women." *Journal of the American Medical Association,* vol. 252 (1984), pp. 487–90.

Boyer, J. L., and F. W. Kasch. "Exercise Therapy in Hypertensive Men." *Journal of the American Medical Association,* vol. 211 (1970), pp. 1668–71.

Brand, R. J., R. S. Paffenbarger, Jr., R. I. Scholtz, and J.B. Kampert. "Work Activity and Fatal Heart Attack Studied by Multiple Logistic Risk Analysis." *American Journal of Epidemiology,* vol. 110 (1979), pp. 52–62.

Caspersen, C. J., K. E. Powell, and G. M. Christenson. "Physical Activity, Exercise, and Physical Fitness: Definitions and Distinctions for Health Related Research." *Public Health Reports,* vol. 100 (1985), pp. 126–31.

Chalmers, J., and K. C. Ho. "Geographical Variations in Senile Osteoporosis: The Association with Physical Activity." *Journal of Bone and Joint Surgery,* vol. 52B (1970), pp. 667–75.

Choquette, G., and R. J. Ferguson. "Blood Pressure Reduction in 'Borderline' Hypertensives Following Physical Training." *Canadian Medical Association Journal,* vol. 108 (1973), pp. 699–703.

Cooper, K. H., M. L. Pollock, R. P. Martin, and others. "Physical Fitness Levels vs. Selected Coronary Risk Factors: A Cross-sectional Study." *Journal of the American Medical Association,* vol. 236 (1976), pp. 166–69.

Dalén, N., and K. E. Olsson. "Bone Mineral Content and Physical Activity." *Acta Orthopaedica Scandinavica,* vol. 45 (1974), pp. 170–74.

Dehn, M. M., and R. A. Bruce. "Longitudinal Variations in Maximal Oxygen Intake with Age and Activity." *Journal of Applied Physiology,* vol. 33 (1972), pp. 805–07.

Drinkwater, B. L., K. Nilson, C. H. Chesnut III, and others. "Bone Mineral Content of Amenorrheic and Eumenorrheic Athletes." *New England Journal of Medicine,* vol. 311 (1984), pp. 277–81.

Duncan, J. J., J. E. Farr, B. Upton, and others. "The Effects of Aerobic Exercise on Plasma Catecholamines and Blood Pressure in Patients with Mild Essential Hypertension." *Journal of the American Medical Association,* vol. 254 (1985), pp. 2609–13.

Epstein, L. H., R. R. Wing, R. Koeske, and others. "A Comparison of Lifestyle Change and Programmed Aerobic Exercise on Weight and Fitness Change in Obese Children." *Behavior Therapy,* vol. 13 (1982), pp. 651–65.

Freedman, L.W. "The Metabolism of Calcium in Patients with Spinal Cord Injury." *Annals of Surgery,* vol. 129 (1949), pp. 177–84.

Garcia-Palmieri, M. R., R. Costas, M. Cruz-Vidal, and others. "Increased Physical Activity: A Protective Factor Against Heart Attacks in Puerto Rico." *American Journal of Cardiology,* vol. 50 (1982), pp. 749–55.

Gibbons, L. W., S. N. Blair, K. H. Cooper, and others. "Association between Coronary Heart Disease Risk Factors and Physical Fitness in Healthy Adult Women." *Circulation*, vol. 67 (1983), pp. 977–83.

Grimby, G., and B. Saltin. "Physiological Analysis of Physically Well-Trained Middle-Aged and Old Athletes." *Acta Medica Scandinavica*, vol. 179 (1966), pp. 513–26.

Hansson, T. H., B. O. Roos, and A. Nachemson. "Development of Osteopenia in the Fourth Lumbar Vertebra During Prolonged Bed Rest After Operation for Scoliosis." *Acta Orthopaedica Scandinavica*, vol. 46 (1975), pp. 621–30.

Haskell, W. L., and S. N. Blair. "The Physical Activity Component of Health Promotion in Occupational Settings." *Public Health Reports*, vol. 95 (1980), pp. 109–18.

Heath, G. W., J. M. Hagberg, A. A. Ehsani, and J. O. Holloszy. "A Physiological Comparison of Young and Older Endurance Athletes." *Journal of Applied Physiology: Environmental and Exercise Physiology*, vol. 51 (1981), pp. 634–40.

Hicky, N., R. Mulcahy, J. Bourke, and others. "Study of Coronary Risk Factors Related to Physical Activity in 15,171 Men." *British Medical Journal*, vol. 3 (1975), pp. 507–09.

King, H., R. Taylor, P. Zimmet, and others. "Non-insulin Dependent Diabetes (NIDDM) in a Newly Independent Pacific Nation: The Republic of Kiribati." *Diabetes Care*, vol. 7 (1984), pp. 409–15.

Koplan, J. P., K. E. Powell, R. K. Sikes, and others. "An Epidemiologic Study of the Benefits and Risks of Running." *Journal of the American Medical Association*, vol. 248 (1982), pp. 3118–21.

Krølner, B., B. Toft, S. P. Nielsen, and others. "Physical Exercise as a Phrophylaxis Against Involuntary Bone Loss: Controlled Trial." *Clinical Science*, vol. 64 (1983), pp. 541–46.

Krølner, B., and B. Toft. "Vertebral Bone Loss: An Unheeded Side Effect of Therapeutic Bed Rest." *Clinical Science*, vol. 64 (1983), pp. 537–40.

Kukkonen, K., R. Rauramaa, E. Voutilainen, and others. "Physical Training of Middle-Aged Men with Borderline Hypertension." *Annals of Clinical Research*, vol. 14, supplement 34 (1982), pp. 139–45.

Lane, N. E., D. A. Bloch, H. H. Jones, and others. "Long-Distance Running, Bone Density, and Osteoarthritis." *Journal of the American Medical Association*, vol. 255 (1986), pp. 1147–51.

Linden, V. "Absence from Work and Physical Fitness." *British Journal of Industrial Medicine*, vol. 26 (1969), pp. 47–53.

Mann, G. V., H. L. Garrett, A. Farhi, and others. "Exercise to Prevent Coronary Heart Disease: An Experimental Study of the Effects of Training on Risk Factors for Coronary Disease in Men." *American Journal of Medicine,* vol. 46 (1969), pp. 12–27.

Mazess, R. B., and G. D. Whedon. "Immobilization and Bone." *Calcified Tissue International,* vol. 35 (1983), pp. 265–67.

Morris J. N., M. G. Everitt, R. Pollard, and others. "Exercise and the Heart (letter to the editor)." *Lancet,* vol. 1 (1981), p. 267.

Morris, J. N., M. G. Everitt, R. Pollard, and S. P. W. Chave. "Vigorous Exercise in Leisure-time: Protection Against Coronary Heart Disease." *Lancet,* vol. 2 (1980), pp. 1207–10.

Paffenbarger, R. S., and W. E. Hale. "Work Activity and Coronary Heart Mortality." *New England Journal of Medicine,* vol. 292 (1975), pp. 545–50.

Paffenbarger, R. S., Jr., R. T. Hyde, and A. L. Wing. "Physical Activity, All-cause Mortality, and Longevity of College Alumni." *New England Journal of Medicine,* vol. 314 (1986), pp. 605–13.

Paffenbarger, R. S., Jr., R. T. Hyde, A. L. Wing, and C. H. Steinmetz. "A Natural History of Athleticism and Cardiovascular Health." *Journal of the American Medical Association,* vol. 252 (1984), pp. 491–95.

Paffenbarger, R. S., Jr., A. L. Wing, and R. T. Hyde. "Physical Activity as an Index of Heart Attack Risk in College Alumni." *American Journal of Epidemiology,* vol. 108 (1978), pp. 161–75.

Paffenbarger, R. S., Jr., A. L. Wing, R. T. Hyde, and D. L. Jung. "Physical Activity and Incidence of Hypertension in College Alumni." *American Journal of Epidemiology,* vol. 117 (1983), pp. 245–57.

Panush, R. S., C. Schmidt, J. R. Caldwell, and others. "Is Running Associated With Degenerative Joint Disease?" *Journal of the American Medical Association,* vol. 255 (1986), pp. 1152-54.

Powell, K. E., H. W. Kohl, C. J. Casperson, and S. N. Blair. "An Epidemiologic Perspective of the Causes of Running Injuries." *Physician and Sports Medicine,* vol. 14 (1986), p. 100–14.

Richter, E. A., N. B. Ruderman, and S. H. Schneider. "Diabetes and Exercise." *American Journal of Medicine,* vol. 70 (1981), pp. 201–09.

Roman, O., A. Camuzzi, E. Villalon, and C. Klenner. "Physical Training Program in Arterial Hypertension: A Long-term Prospective Follow-up." *Cardiology,* vol. 67 (1981), pp. 230–43.

Salonen, J. T., P. Puska, and J. Tuomilehto. "Physical Activity and Risk of Myocardial Infarction, Cerebral Stroke and Death: A Longitudinal

Study in Eastern Finland." *American Journal of Epidemiology,* vol. 115 (1982), pp. 526–37.

Shephard, R. J., M. Cox, and P. Corey. "Fitness Program Participation: Its Effect on Worker Performance." *Journal of Occupational Medicine,* vol. 23 (1981), pp. 359–63.

Siscovick, D. S., N. S. Weiss, R. H. Fletcher, and T. Lasky. "The Incidence of Primary Cardiac Arrest During Vigorous Exercise." *New England Journal of Medicine,* vol. 311 (1984), pp. 874–77.

Siscovick, D. S., N. S. Weiss, R. H. Fletcher, and others. "Habitual Vigorous Exercise and Primary Cardiac Arrest: Effect of Other Risk Factors on the Relationship." *Journal of Chronic Diseases,* vol. 37 (1984), pp. 625–31.

Siscovick, D. S., N. S. Weiss, A. P. Hallstrom, and others. "Physical Activity and Primary Cardiac Arrest." *Journal of the American Medical Association,* vol. 248 (1982), pp. 3113–17.

Stamler, J., E. Farinaro, L. M. Mojonnier, and others. "Prevention and Control of Hypertension by Nutritional-Hygienic Means: Long-term Experience of the Chicago Coronary Prevention Evaluation Program." *Journal of the American Medical Association,* vol. 243 (1980), pp. 1819–23.

Stein, H., S. Sabato, I. Leichter, and others. " A New Method of Measuring Bone Density in the Lower Tibia of Normal and Post Injury Limbs: A Quantitative and Comparative Study." *Clinical Orthopaedics and Related Research,* vol. 174 (1983), pp. 181–87.

Taylor, C. B., J. F. Sallis, and R. Needle. "The Relation of Physical Activity and Exercise to Mental Health." *Public Health Reports,* vol. 100 (1985), pp. 195–202.

Whedon, D.G., and E. Shorr. "Metabolic Studies in Paralytic Acute Anterior Poliomyelitis: Alterations in Calcium and Phosphorous Metabolism." *Journal of Clinical Investigation,* vol. 36 (1957), pp. 966–81.

Zimmet, P., S. Faaiuso, J. Ainuu, and others. "The Prevalence of Diabetes in the Rural and Urban Polynesian Population of Western Samoa." *Diabetes,* vol. 30 (1981), pp. 45–51.

Dietary Calcium

Alevizaki, C. C., D. G. Ikkos, and P. Singhelakis. "Progressive Decrease of True Intestinal Calcium Absorption with Age in Normal Man." *Journal of Nuclear Medicine,* vol. 14 (1973), pp. 760–62.

Alffram, P. A., and G. C. H. Bauer. "Epidemiology of Fractures of the Forearm: A Biomechanical Investigation of Bone Strength." *Journal of Bone and Joint Surgery,* vol. 44A (1962), pp. 105–14.

Avioli, L. V., J. E. McDonald, and S. W. Lee. "The Influence of Age on the Intestinal Absorption of [47]Ca in Women and Its Relation to [47]Ca Absorption in Postmenopausal Osteoporosis." *Journal of Clinical Investigation,* vol. 44 (1965), pp. 1960–67.

Barkin, J., D. R. Wilson, M. A. Manuel, and others. "Bone Mineral Content in Idiopathic Calcium Nephrolithiasis." *Mineral and Electrolyte Metabolism,* vol. 11 (1985), pp. 19–24.

Belizan, J. M., J. Villar, O. Pineda, and others. "Reduction of Blood Pressure with Calcium Supplementation in Young Adults." *Journal of the American Medical Association,* vol. 249 (1983), pp. 1161–65.

Bernstein, D. S., N. Sadowsky, D. M. Hegsted, and others. "Prevalence of Osteoporosis in High- and Low-Fluoride Areas in North Dakota." *Journal of the American Medical Association,* vol. 198 (1966), pp. 499–504.

Bullamore, J. R., J. C. Gallagher, R. Wilkinson, and others. "Effect of Age on Calcium Absorption." *Lancet,* vol. 2 (1970), pp. 535–37.

Caniggia, A., C. Gennari, V. Bianchi, and others. "Intestinal Absorption of [45]Ca in Senile Osteoporosis." *Acta Medica Scandinavica,* vol. 173 (1963), pp. 613–17.

Consensus Conference. "Osteoporosis." *Journal of the American Medical Association,* vol. 252 (1984), pp. 799–802.

Cummings, S. R., J. L. Kelsey, M. C. Nevitt, and others. "Epidemiology of Osteoporosis and Osteoporotic Fractures." *Epidemiologic Reviews,* vol. 7 (1985), pp. 178–208.

Dent, C. E., H. E. Engelbrecht, and R.C. Godfrey. "Osteoporosis of Lumbar Vertebrae and Calcification of Abdominal Aorta in Women Living in Durban." *British Medical Journal,* vol. 4 (1968), pp. 76–79.

Fujita, T., Y. Okamoto, Y. Sakagami, and others. "Bone Changes and Aortic Calcification in Aging Inhabitants of Mountain versus Seacoast Communities in the Kii Peninsula." *Journal of the American Geriatrics Society,* vol. 32 (1984), pp. 124–28.

Gallagher, J. C., J. Aaron, A. Horsman, and others. "The Crush Fracture Syndrome in Postmenopausal Women." *Clinics in Endocrinology and Metabolism,* vol. 2 (1973), pp. 293–315.

Gallagher, J. C., C. M. Jerpbak, W. S. S. Jee, and others. "1,25-dihydroxyvitamin D_3: Short- and Long-Term Effects on Bone and Calcium Metabolism in Patients with Postmenopausal Osteoporosis." *Proceedings of the National Academy of Sciences of the United States of America: Biological Sciences,* vol. 79 (1982), pp. 3325–29.

Gallagher, J. C., B. L. Riggs, J. Eisman, and others. "Intestinal Calcium Absorption and Serum Vitamin D Metabolites in Normal Subjects and Osteoporotic Patients: Effect of Age and Dietary Calcium." *Journal of Clinical Investigation,* vol. 64 (1979), pp. 729–36.

Garland, C. F., and F. C. Garland. "Do Sunlight and Vitamin D Reduce the Likelihood of Colon Cancer?" *International Journal of Epidemiology,* vol. 9 (1980), pp. 227–31.

Garland, C., R. B. Shekelle, E. Barrett-Connor, and others. "Dietary Vitamin D and Calcium and Risk of Colorectal Cancer: A 19-year Prospective Study in Men." *Lancet,* vol. 1 (1985), pp. 307–09.

Haupt, B. J., and E. Graves. *Detailed Diagnoses and Surgical Procedures for Patients Discharged from Short-Stay Hospitals, United States, 1979.* DHHS (PHS) 81-1274-1. Washington, D.C.: Department of Health and Human Services, 1982.

Heaney, R. P. "Calcium, Bone Health and Osteoporosis." In *Bone and Mineral Research: A Yearly Survey of Developments in the Field of Bone and Mineral Metabolism,* vol. 4, edited by W. A. Peck. Amsterdam: Elsevier, 1985.

Heaney, R. P., J. C. Gallagher, C. C. Johnston, and others. "Calcium Nutrition and Bone Health in the Elderly." *American Journal of Clinical Nutrition,* vol. 36 (1982), pp. 986–1013.

Heaney, R. P., R. R. Recker, and P. D. Saville. "Calcium Balance and Calcium Requirements in Middle-Aged Women." *American Journal of Clinical Nutrition,* vol. 30 (1977), pp. 1603–11.

———. "Menopausal Changes in Calcium Balance Performance." *Journal of Laboratory and Clinical Medicine,* vol. 92 (1978), pp. 953–63.

Heaney, R. P., P. D. Saville, and R. R. Recker. "Calcium Absorption as a Function of Calcium Intake." *Journal of Laboratory and Clinical Medicine,* vol. 85 (1975), pp. 881–90.

Horowitz, M., A. G. Need, J. C. Philcox, and others. "Effect of Calcium Supplementation on Urinary Hydroxyproline in Osteoporotic Postmenopausal Women." *American Journal of Clinical Nutrition,* vol. 39 (1984), pp. 857–59.

Horsman, A., J. C. Gallagher, M. Simpson, and B. E. C. Nordin. "Prospective Trial of Oestrogen and Calcium in Postmenopausal Women." *British Medical Journal,* vol. 2 (1977), pp. 789–92.

Ireland, P., and J. S. Fordtran. "Effect of Dietary Calcium and Age on Jejunal Calcium Absorption in Humans Studied by Intestinal Perfusion." *Journal of Clinical Investigation,* vol. 52 (1973), pp. 2672–81.

Iskrant, A. P., and R. W. Smith, Jr. "Osteoporosis in Women 45 Years and Over Related to Subsequent Fractures." *Public Health Reports,* vol. 84 (1969), pp. 33–38.

Johnston, C. C., Jr. "Studies on the Prevention of Age-Related Bone Loss." In *Bone and Mineral Research: A Yearly Survey of Developments in the Field of Bone and Mineral Metabolism,* vol. 3, edited by W. A. Peck. Amsterdam: Elsevier, 1985.

Johnston, C. C., Jr., and S. Epstein. "Clinical, Biochemical, Radiographic, Epidemiologic and Economic Features of Osteoporosis." *Orthopedic Clinics of North America,* vol. 12 (1981), pp. 559–69.

Johnson, N. E., E. L. Smith, and J. L. Freudenheim. "Effects on Blood Pressure of Calcium Supplementation of Women." *American Journal of Clinical Nutrition,* vol. 42 (1985), pp. 12–17.

Jowsey, J., and J. Gershon-Cohen. "Effect of Dietary Calcium Levels on Production and Reversal of Experimental Osteoporosis in Cats." *Proceedings of the Society for Experimental Biology and Medicine,* vol. 116 (1964), pp. 437–41.

Keene, J. S., and C. A. Anderson. "Hip Fractures in the Elderly: Discharge Predictions with a Functional Rating Scale." *Journal of the American Medical Association,* vol. 248 (1982), pp. 564–67.

Kleerekoper, M., A. M. Parfitt, and B. I. Ellis. "Measurement of Vertebral Fracture Rates in Osteoporosis." In *Osteoporosis: Proceedings of the Copenhagen Symposium on Osteoporosis, June 3–8, 1984,* edited by C. Christiansen, C. D. Arnaud, B. E. C. Nordin and others. Denmark: Department of Clinical Chemistry, Glostrup Hospital, 1984.

Knapp, E. L. "Factors Influencing the Urinary Excretion of Calcium." *Journal of Clinical Investigation,* vol. 26 (1947), pp. 182–202.

Lewinnek, G. E., J. E. Kelsey, A. A. White III, and others. "The Significance and Comparative Analysis of the Epidemiology of Hip Fractures." *Clinical Orthopedics and Related Research,* vol. 152 (1980), pp. 35–43.

Lipkin, M., and H. Newmark. "Effect of Added Dietary Calcium on Colonic Epithelial-Cell Proliferation in Subjects at High Risk for Familial Colonic Cancer." *New England Journal of Medicine,* vol. 313 (1985), pp. 1381–84.

Lutwak, L., and G. D. Whedon. "Osteoporosis." *Disease-A-Month* (April 1963), pp. 1–39.

Matkovic, V., K. Kostial, I. Simonovic, and others. "Bone Status and Fracture Rates in Two Regions of Yugoslavia." *American Journal of Clinical Nutrition,* vol. 32 (1979), pp. 540–49.

McCarron, D. A., and C. D. Morris. "Blood Pressure Response to Oral Calcium in Persons with Mild to Moderate Hypertension: A Randomized, Double-Blind, Placebo-Controlled, Crossover Trial." *Annals of Internal Medicine,* vol. 103 (1985), pp. 825–31.

Newcomer, A. D., S. F. Hodgson, D. B. McGill, and others. "Lactase Deficiency: Prevalence in Osteoporosis." *Annals of Internal Medicine,* vol. 89 (1978), pp. 218–20.

Nilas, L., C. Christiansen, and P. Rødbro. "Calcium Supplementation and Postmenopausal Bone Loss." *British Medical Journal,* vol. 289 (1984), pp. 1103–06

Nordin, B. E. C. "Osteomalacia, Osteoporosis, and Calcium Deficiency." *Clinical Orthopaedics,* vol. 17 (1960), pp. 235–58.

Nordin, B. E. C., A. Horsman, R. G. Crilly, and others. "Treatment of Spinal Osteoporosis in Postmenopausal Women." *British Medical Journal,* vol. 280 (1980), pp. 451–54.

Nordin, B. E. C., R. Wilkinson, D. H. Marshall, and others. "Calcium Absorption in the Elderly." *Calcified Tissue Research,* vol. 21 (1976), pp. 442-51.

Owen, R. A., L. J. Melton III, K. A. Johnson, and others. "Incidence of Colles' Fracture in a North American Community." *American Journal of Public Health,* vol. 72 (1982), pp. 605–07.

Pacifici, R., D. Droke, and L. V. Avioli. "Comment: Intestinal Lactase Activity and Calcium Absorption in the Aging Female with Osteoporosis." *Calcified Tissue International,* vol. 37 (1985), pp. 101–02.

Parfitt, A. M., J. C. Gallagher, R. P. Heaney, and others. "Vitamin D and Bone Health in the Elderly." *American Journal of Clinical Nutrition,* vol. 36 (1982), pp. 1014–31.

Phillips, R. L. "Role of Life-Style and Dietary Habits in Risk of Cancer Among Seventh Day Adventists." *Cancer Research,* vol. 35 (1975), pp. 3513–22.

Recker, R. R., and R. P. Heaney. "The Effect of Milk Supplements on

Calcium Metabolism, Bone Metabolism and Calcium Balance." *American Journal of Clinical Nutrition*, vol. 41 (1985), pp. 254–63.

Recker, R. R., P. D. Saville, and R. P. Heaney. "Effect of Estrogens and Calcium Carbonate on Bone Loss in Postmenopausal Women." *Annals of Internal Medicine*, vol. 87 (1977), pp. 649–55.

Reed, D., D. McGee, K. Yano, and others. "Diet, Blood Pressure and Multicollinearity." *Hypertension*, vol. 7 (1985), pp. 405–10.

Riggs, B. L., E. Seeman, S. F. Hodgson, and others. "Effect of the Fluoride/Calcium Regimen on Vertebral Fracture Occurrence in Postmenopausal Osteoporosis." *New England Journal of Medicine*, vol. 306 (1982), pp. 446–50.

Riggs, B. L., H. W. Wahner, W. L. Dunn, and others. "Differential Changes in Bone Mineral Density of the Appendicular and Axial Skeleton with Aging." *Journal of Clinical Investigation*, vol. 67 (1981), pp. 328–35.

Rivlin, R. S. "Nutrition and Osteoporosis." *Public Health Reports*, forthcoming.

Robertson, W. G., M. Peacock, and A. Hodgkinson. "Dietary Changes and the Incidence of Urinary Calculi in the U.K. between 1958 and 1976." *Journal of Chronic Diseases*, vol. 32 (1979), pp. 469–76.

Sakhaee, K., M. Nicar, K. Glass, and others. "Reduction in Intestinal Calcium Absorption by Hydrochlorothiazide in Postmenopausal Osteoporosis." *Journal of Clinical Endocrinology and Metabolism*, vol. 59 (1984), pp. 1037–42.

Shah, B. G., G. V. G. Krishnarao, and H. H. Draper. "The Relationship of Ca and P Nutrition during Adult Life and Osteoporosis in Aged Mice." *Journal of Nutrition*, vol. 92 (1967), pp. 30–34.

Snedeker, S. M., S. A. Smith, and J. L. Greger. "Effect of Dietary Calcium and Phosphorus Levels on the Utilization of Iron, Copper, and Zinc by Adult Males." *Journal of Nutrition*, vol. 112 (1982), pp. 136–43.

Teppo, L., and E. Saxén. "Epidemiology of Colon Cancer in Scandinavia." *Israel Journal of Medical Sciences*, vol. 15 (1979), pp. 322–28.

Thallassinos, N.C., D. H. Gutteridge, G. F. Joplin, and others. "Calcium Balance in Osteoporotic Patients on Long-Term Oral Calcium Therapy with and without Sex Hormones." *Clinical Science*, vol. 62 (1982), pp. 221–26.

Transbøl, I., M. S. Christensen, G. F. Jensen, and others. "Thiazide for the Postponement of Postmenopausal Bone Loss." *Metabolism: Clinical and Experimental,* vol. 31 (1982), pp. 383–86.

Wasnich, R. D., R. J. Benfante, K. Yano, and others. "Thiazide Effect on the Mineral Content of Bone." *New England Journal of Medicine,* vol. 309 (1983), pp. 344–47.

Weiss, N. S., J. M. Liff, C. L. Ure, and others. "Mortality in Women Following Hip Fracture." *Journal of Chronic Diseases,* vol. 36 (1983), pp. 879–82.

Wical, K. E., and P. Brussee. "Effects of a Calcium and Vitamin D Supplement on Alveolar Ridge Resorption in Immediate Denture Patients." *Journal of Prosthetic Dentistry,* vol. 41 (1979), pp. 4–11.

Yano, K., L. K. Heilbrun, R. D. Wasnich, and others. "The Relationship between Diet and Bone Mineral Content of Multiple Skeletal Sites in Elderly Japanese-American Men and Women Living in Hawaii. *American Journal of Clinical Nutrition,* vol. 42 (1985), pp. 877–88.

Alcohol Use

Alibrandi, T. *Young Alcoholics.* Minneapolis, Minn.: Comp Care, 1978.

Baekeland, F., L. Lundwall, and B. Kissin. "Methods for the Treatment of Chronic Alcoholism: A Critical Appraisal." In *Research Advances in Alcohol and Drug Problems,* vol. 2, edited by Y. Israel. New York: John Wiley and Sons, 1975.

Brandsma, J. M. *Outpatient Treatment of Alcoholism: A Review and Comparative Study.* Baltimore: University Park Press, 1980.

Burnett, J. "Pursuing Safety Across All Modes." Keynote address at the Transportation Workshop on Performance Guidelines Related to Alcohol and Other Drugs, sponsored by the American Automobile Association, Washington, D.C., January 16–17, 1986.

Cook, P. J. "The Effect of Liquor Taxes on Drinking, Cirrhosis, and Auto Accidents." In *Alcohol and Public Policy: Beyond the Shadow of Prohibition,* edited by M. H. Moore and D. R. Gernstein, pp. 255–85. Washington, D.C.: National Academy Press, 1981.

Cook, P. J., and G. Tauchen. "The Effect of Liquor Taxes on Heavy Drinking." *Bell Journal of Economics,* vol. 13 (1982), pp. 379–90.

Costello, R. M. "Evaluation of Alcoholism Treatment Programs." In *Encyclopedic Handbook of Alcoholism,* edited by E. M. Pattison and E. Kaufman. New York: Gardner Press, 1982.

Cucchiaro, S., J. Ferreira, Jr., and A. Sicherman. *The Effect of the 18-Year-Old Drinking Age on Auto Accidents.* Cambridge, Mass.: Massachusetts Institute of Technology, Operations Research Center, 1974.

Douglass, R. L., and J. A. Freedman. *Alcohol-related Casualties and Alcohol Beverage Market Response to Beverage Alcohol Availability Policies in Michigan.* Ann Arbor: The University of Michigan, Highway Safety Research Institute, 1977.

Emrick, C. D. "A Review of Psychologically Oriented Treatment of Alcoholism: The Use and Interrelationships of Outcome Criteria and Drinking Behavior Following Treatment." *Quarterly Journal of Studies on Alcohol,* vol. 35 (1974), pp. 523–49.

Emrick, C. D. "Evaluation of Alcoholism Therapy Methods." In *Encyclopedic Handbook of Alcoholism,* edited by E. M. Pattison and E. Kaufman. New York: Gardner Press, 1982.

Fell, J. C. *Alcohol Involvement in United States Traffic Accidents: Where It Is Changing.* Washington, D.C.: National Highway Traffic Safety Administration, 1983.

Fell, J. C., and B.G. Hazzard. "The Role of Alcohol Involvement in Fatal Pedestrian Collisions." *Proceedings of the 29th Conference of the American Association for Automotive Medicine, October 7–9, 1985,* pp. 105–25. Washington, D.C., AAAM, 1985.

Filkins, L. D., and J. D. Flora. *Alcohol-related Accidents and DUI Arrests in Michigan: 1978–1979.* Ann Arbor: The University of Michigan, Highway Safety Research Institute, 1981.

Goodwin, D. W. *Alcoholism: The Facts.* New York: Oxford University Press, 1981.

Graham, G. Statement. In U.S. Senate, Committee on Finance, Subcommittee on Health. *Medicare Coverage of Alcoholism Treatment.* Hearing, 97 Cong. 2 sess. Washington, D.C.: Government Printing Office, 1982.

Grossman, M. "Price Sensitivity and Teenage Alcoholic Beverage Consumption." Paper presented at the 113th Annual Meeting of the American Public Health Association, Washington, D.C., November 17–21, 1985.

Grossman, M., D. Coate, and G.M. Arluck. "Price Sensitivity of Alcoholic Beverages in the United States." In *Control Issues in Alcohol Abuse Prevention: Strategies for States and Communities,* edited by H. D. Holder. Greenwich, Conn.: JAI Press, forthcoming.

Hill, M. J., and H. T. Blane. "Evaluation of Psychotherapy with Alcoholics." *Quarterly Journal of Studies in Alcohol,* vol. 28 (1967), pp. 76–104.

Hingson, R., N. Scotch, T. Mangione, and others. "Impact of Legislation Raising the Legal Drinking Age in Massachusetts from 18 to 20." *American Journal of Public Health,* vol. 73 (1983), pp. 163–70.

Hoadley, J. F., B. C. Fuchs, and H. D. Holder. "The Effect of Alcohol Beverage Restrictions on Consumption: A 25-Year Longitudinal Analysis." *American Journal of Drug and Alcohol Abuse,* vol.10 (1984), pp. 375–401.

Holder, H. D. "Alcoholism Treatment and Health Care Utilization and Costs: Potential for 'Offset' Reductions." *Medical Care,* vol. 25 (1987), pp. 52–71.

Klein, T. M. *The Effect of Raising the Minimum Legal Drinking Age on Traffic Accidents in the State of Maine.* DOT HS-806-149. Washington, D.C.: National Highway Traffic Safety Administration, 1981.

Klerman, G. L. "Prevention of Alcoholism." In *Prevention of Alcoholism,* edited by J. Solomon. New York: Plenum Press, 1982.

Levy, D., and N. Sheflin. "The Demand for Alcoholic Beverages: An Aggregate Time-Series Analysis for the United States." Center of Alcohol Studies, Rutgers University, New Brunswick, N. J., 1981.

Lillis, R. P., T. P. Williams, and W. R. Williford. "The Impact of the 19-Year-Old Drinking Age in New York." In *Control Issues in Alcohol Abuse Prevention: Strategies for States and Communities,* edited by H. D. Holder. Greenwich, Conn.: JAI Press, forthcoming.

Luna, G. K., R. V. Maier, L. Sowder, and others. "The Influence of Ethanol Intoxication on Outcome of Injured Motorcyclists." *Journal of Trauma,* vol. 24 (1984), pp. 695–700.

Lynn, C. *The Effects of Lowering the Legal Drinking Age in Virginia: Final Report.* Charlottesville, Va.: Virginia Highway and Transportation Research Council, 1981.

Manisses Communications Group. *The Alcoholism Report: The Authoritative Newsletter for Professionals in the Field of Alcoholism,* July 30, 1986.

McCrady, B. S., and K. J. Shear. "Alcoholism Treatment Approaches: Patient Variables, Treatment Variables." In *Medical and Social Aspects of Alcohol Use,* edited by B. Tabakoff, P. B. Sutker, and C. L. Randall. New York: Plenum Press, 1983.

Medhus, A. "Mortality Among Female Alcoholics." *Scandinavian Journal of Social Medicine,* vol. 3 (1975), p. 111–15.

Ornstein, I., and D. M. Hanssens. "Alcohol Control Laws, Consumer

Welfare, and the Demand for Distilled Spirits and Beer." Working Paper 102. Graduate School of Management, UCLA, 1981.

Saxe, L., D. Dougherty, K. Esty, and M. Fine. *The Effectiveness and Costs of Alcoholism Treatment.* OTA-HCS-22-P. U.S. Congress, Office of Technology Assessment. Government Printing Office, 1983.

Smith, R. A., R. W. Hingson, S. Morelock, and others. "Legislation Raising the Legal Drinking Age in Massachusetts from 18 to 20: Effect on 16 and 17 Year Olds." *Journal of Studies on Alcohol,* vol. 45 (1984), pp. 534–39.

U.S. National Highway Traffic Safety Administration. *Evaluation of Minimum Drinking Age Laws Using the National Electronic Injury Surveillance System.* DOT-HS-806-097. Washington, D.C.: NHTSA, 1982.

U.S. National Transportation Safety Board. *Safety Study: Recreational Boating Safety and Alcohol.* NTSB no. SS-83-02. NTIS no. PB83-917006. Washington, D.C.: NTSB, 1983.

U. S. Public Health Service. *Healthy People: The Surgeon General's Report on Health Promotion and Disease Prevention.* DHEW 79-55071. Washington, D.C.: Department of Health, Education, and Welfare, 1979.

U.S. Public Health Service, Alcohol, Drug Abuse, and Mental Health Administration. *Fifth Special Report to the U.S. Congress on Alcohol and Health from the Secretary of Health and Human Services.* DHHS (ADM) 84-1291. Washington, D.C.: Department of Health and Human Services, 1984.

Vaillant, G.E. *The Natural History of Alcoholism.* Cambridge: Harvard University Press, 1983.

Voas, R.B., and J. Moulden. "Alcohol Use and Driving by Young Americans." In *Minimum-Drinking-Age Laws: An Evaluation,* edited by H. Wechsler. Lexington, Mass.: Lexington Books, 1980.

Voegtlin, W. L., and F. Lemere, "The Treatment of Alcohol Addiction: A Review of the Literature." *Quarterly Journal of Studies on Alcohol,* vol. 2 (1942), pp. 717–803.

Wagenaar, A. C. *Alcohol, Young Drivers, and Traffic Accidents: Effects of Minimum-Age Laws.* Lexington, Mass.: Lexington Books, 1983.

Wagenaar, A. C. "Effects of Minimum Drinking Age on Alcohol-Related Traffic Crashes: The Michigan Experience Five Years Later." In *Control Issues in Alcohol Abuse Prevention: Strategies for States and Communities,* edited by H. D. Holder. Greenwich, Conn.: JAI Press, forthcoming.

Waller, P. F., A. R. Hansen, J. C. Stutts, and C. L. Popkin. "Alcohol: A

Potentiating Factor in Motor Vehicle Crash Injury." SAE Technical Paper Series. Warrendale, Pa.: Society of Automotive Engineers, 1986.

Williams, A. F., P. L. Zador, S. S. Harris, and R. S. Karpf. "The Effect of Raising the Legal Minimum Drinking Age on Fatal Crash Involvement." Washington, D.C.: Insurance Institute for Highway Safety, 1981.

————. "The Effect of Raising the Legal Minimum Drinking Age on Involvement in Fatal Crashes." *Journal of Legal Studies,* vol. 12 (1983), pp. 169–79.

Obesity

Abraham, S., G. Collins, and M. Nordsieck. "Relationship of Childhood Weight Status to Morbidity in Adults." *Health Services and Mental Health Administration Health Reports,* vol. 86 (1971), pp. 273–84.

Andres, R., D. Elahi, J. D. Tobin, and others. "Impact of Age on Weight Goals." *Annals of Internal Medicine,* vol. 103 (1985), pp. 1030–33.

Ashley, F. W., Jr., and W. B. Kannel. "Relation of Weight Change to Changes in Atherogenic Traits." *Journal of Chronic Diseases,* vol. 27 (1974), pp. 103–14.

Bray, G. A., ed. *Obesity in Perspective, Part One,* vol. 2. DHEW (NIH) 75–708. Washington, D.C.: Department of Health, Education, and Welfare (HEW), 1976.

————, ed. *Obesity in America: A Conference.* DHEW (NIH) 79-359. Washington, D.C.: HEW, 1979.

————. *Obesity.* Kalamazoo, Mich.: Upjohn, 1982.

————. "Obesity—A Disease of Nutrient or Energy Balance?" *Nutrition Reviews,* vol. 45 (1987), pp. 33–43.

Drenick, E. J., G. S. Bale, F. Seltzer, and D. G. Johnson. "Excessive Mortality and Causes of Death in Morbidly Obese Men." *Journal of the American Medical Association,* vol. 243 (1980), pp. 443–45.

Dustan, H. P. "Obesity and Hypertension." *Annals of Internal Medicine,* vol. 103 (1985), pp. 1047–49.

Feinleib, M. "Epidemiology of Obesity in Relation to Health Hazards." *Annals of Internal Medicine,* vol. 103 (1985), pp. 1019–24.

Goldblatt, P. B., M. E. Moore, and A. J. Stunkard. "Social Factors in Obesity." *Journal of the American Medical Association,* vol. 192 (1965), p. 1039.

Hubert, H. B., N. Feinleib, P. McNamara, and W. P. Castelli. "Obesity as an Independent Risk Factor for Cardiovascular Disease: A Twenty-six-year Follow-up of Participants in the Framingham Heart Study." *Circulation*, vol. 67 (1983), pp. 968–77.

Kannel, W. B., and T. Gordon. "Physiological and Medical Concomitants of Obesity: The Framingham Study." In *Obesity in America: A Conference*, edited by G. A. Bray, pp. 125–63. DHEW (NIH) 79-359. Washington, D.C.: HEW, 1979.

Kissebah, A. H., N. Vydelingum, R. Murray, and others. "Relation of Body Fat Distribution to Metabolic Complications of Obesity." *Journal of Clinical Endocrinology and Metabolism*, vol. 54 (1982), pp. 254–60.

Lapidus, L., C. Bengtsson, B. Larsson, and others. "Distribution of Adipose Tissue and Risk of Cardiovascular Disease and Death: A 12-Year Follow-up of Participants in the Population Study of Women in Gothenberg, Sweden." *British Medical Journal*, vol. 289 (1984), pp. 1257–61.

Larsson, B., P. Björntorp, and G. Tibblin. "The Health Consequences of Moderate Obesity." *International Journal of Obesity*, vol. 5 (1981), pp. 97–116.

Larsson, B., K. Svärdsudd, L. Welin, and others. "Abdominal Adipose Tissue Distribution, Obesity, and Risk of Cardiovascular Disease and Death: 13-Year Follow-up of Participants in the Population Study of Men Born in 1913." *British Medical Journal*, vol. 288 (1984), pp. 1401–04.

Lew, E. A., and L. Garfinkel. "Variations in Mortality by Weight Among 750,000 Men and Women." *Journal of Chronic Diseases*, vol. 32 (1979), pp. 563–76.

Metropolitan Life Insurance Co. "New Weight Standards for Men and Women." *Statistical Bulletin: Metropolitan Life Insurance*, vol. 40 (1959), pp. 1–10.

The Pooling Project Research Group. "Relationship of Blood Pressure, Serum Cholesterol, Smoking Habits, Relative Weight, and ECG Abnormalities to Incidence of Major Coronary Events: Final Report of the Pooling Project." *Journal of Chronic Diseases*, vol. 31 (1978), pp. 201—306.

Reisin, E., R. Abel, M. Modan, and others. "Effect of Weight Loss without Salt Restriction on Reduction of Blood Pressure in Overweight Hyptertension Patients." *New England Journal of Medicine*, vol. 298 (1978), pp. 1–6.

Society of Actuaries, and Society of Life Insurance Medical Directors. *Build Study of 1979*. Society of Actuaries and Society of Life Insurance Medical Directors of America, Itasca, Ill., 1979.

Sohar, E., and E. Sneh. "Follow-Up of Obese Patients: Fourteen Years after a Successful Reducing Diet." *American Journal of Clinical Nutrition,* vol. 26 (1973), pp 845–48.

Stunkard, A. J., "Anorectic Agents Lower Body Weight Set Point." *Life Sciences,* vol. 30 (1982), pp. 2043–55.

Stunkard, A. J., G. D. Foster, and R. F. Grossman. "Surgical Treatment of Obesity." *Advances in Psychosomatic Medicine,* vol. 15 (1986), pp. 144–66.

Stunkard, A. J., and S. B. Penick. "Behavior Modification in the Treatment of Obesity." *Archives of General Psychiatry,* vol. 36 (1979), pp. 801–06.

Stunkard, A. J., J. L. Stinnett, and J. W. Smoller. "Psychological and Social Aspects of the Surgical Treatment of Obesity." *American Journal of Psychiatry,* vol. 143 (1986), pp. 417–29.

Toeller, M., F. A. Gries, and K. Dannehl. "Natural History of Glucose Intolerance in Obesity. A Ten Year Observation." *International Journal of Obesity,* vol. 6, supplement 1 (1982), pp. 145–49.

Tuck, M. L., J. Sowers, L. Dornfeld, and others. "The Effect of Weight Reduction on Blood Pressure, Plasma Renin Activity, and Plasma Aldosterone Levels in Obese Patients." *New England Journal of Medicine,* vol. 304 (1981), pp. 930–33.

U.S. National Center for Health Statistics. Unpublished data from the National Health and Nutrition Examination Survey, 1976–80.

———. *Obese and Overweight Adults in the United States.* Vital and Health Statistics. Series 11, no. 230, DHHS (PHS) 83-1680. Washington, D.C.: Department of Health and Human Services, 1983.

U.S. National Institutes of Health. *Report of the Hypertension Task Force,* vol. 9. DHEW (NIH) 79-1631. Washington, D.C.: HEW, 1979.

———. *Health Implications of Obesity: National Institutes of Health Consensus Development Conference.* Philadelphia, Pa.: American College of Physicians, 1985.

Waaler, H. Th. "Height, Weight and Mortality: The Norwegian Experience." *Acta Medica Scandinavica,* Supplement 679 (1983), pp. 1–56.

Yates, B. T., "Improving the Cost-Effectiveness of Obesity Programs: Three Basic Strategies for Reducing the Cost per Pound." *International Journal of Obesity,* vol. 2 (1978), pp. 249–66.

Yates, B. T., "Cognitive vs. Diet vs. Exercise Components in Obesity Bibliotherapy: Effectiveness as a Function of Psychological Benefits versus Psychological Costs." *Southern Psychologist,* forthcoming.

Guidelines for Cost-Effectiveness Evaluations

Berwick, D. M., and A. L. Komaroff. "Cost Effectiveness of Lead Screening." *New England Journal of Medicine,* vol. 306 (1982), pp. 1392–98.

Cretin, S. "Cost/Benefit Analysis of Treatment and Prevention of Myocardial Infarction." *Health Services Research,* vol. 12 (1977), pp. 174–89.

Kaplan, R. M., J. W. Bush, and C. C. Berry. "The Reliability, Stability, and Generalizability of a Health Status Index." In American Statistical Association, *Proceedings of the Social Statistics Section,* pp. 704–09. Washington, D.C.: ASA, 1978.

Russell, L. B. *Is Prevention Better Than Cure?* Washington, D.C.: Brookings, 1986.

Weinstein, M. C., and W. B. Stason. *Hypertension: A Policy Perspective.* Cambridge: Harvard University Press, 1976.

Workshop Participants

Michele C. Adler, M.P.H.
Head, Retirement Studies
Office for Income Security Policy
Office of the Assistant Secretary for Planning and Evaluation
Department of Health and Human Services

Marilyn Bergner, Ph.D.
Professor of Health Policy and Management
Health Services Research and Development Center
School of Hygiene and Public Health
The Johns Hopkins University

Henry Blackburn, M.D.
Professor and Director, Division of Epidemiology
School of Public Health
University of Minnesota

George A. Bray, M.D.
Professor of Medicine, Physiology, and Biophysics
Chief of Section, Diabetes and Clinical Nutrition
University of Southern California

Jeffrey A. Cutler, M.D.
Medical Officer, Clinical Trials Branch
Division of Epidemiology and Clinical Applications
National Heart, Lung, and Blood Institute
National Institutes of Health

Virginia L. Ernster, Ph.D.
Associate Professor of Epidemiology
School of Medicine
University of California, San Francisco

Donald W. Goodwin, M.D.
Professor and Chairman, Department of Psychiatry
Kansas University Medical Center

Thomas A. Hodgson, Ph.D.
Chief Economist
Office of Analysis and Epidemiology
National Center for Health Statistics
Department of Health and Human Services

John H. Holbrook, M.D.
Associate Professor of Internal Medicine
University of Utah School of Medicine

Harold D. Holder, Ph.D.
Senior Scientist
The Human Ecology Institute, Chapel Hill
Director, Prevention Research Center
Berkeley, California

Robert M. Kaplan, Ph.D.
Professor, Department of Community and Family Medicine
University of California, San Diego

Stephen MacMahon, Ph.D.
Overseas Research Fellow, National Heart Foundation of Australia
Guest Researcher, Clinical Trials Branch
Division of Epidemiology and Clinical Applications
National Heart, Lung, and Blood Institute
National Institutes of Health

Kenneth G. Manton, Ph.D.
Research Professor of Demographic Studies
Duke University Medical Research Professor, Community
   and Family Medicine
Duke University Medical Center

Gerry Oster, Ph.D.
Senior Economist
Policy Analysis, Inc.

Donald L. Patrick, Ph.D., MSPH
Associate Professor
Department of Social and Administrative Medicine
University of North Carolina at Chapel Hill

William A. Peck, M.D.
Simon Professor and Co-Chairman, Department of Medicine
Washington University School of Medicine
Physician-in-Chief
The Jewish Hospital of St. Louis

Kenneth E. Powell, M.D., M.P.H.
Chief, Behavioral Epidemiology and Evaluation Branch
Division of Health Education
Center for Health Promotion and Education
Centers for Disease Control
Department of Health and Human Services

Alice M. Rivlin, Ph.D.
Director, Economic Studies Program
The Brookings Institution

Richard S. Rivlin, M.D.
Chief, Nutrition Service
Memorial Sloan-Kettering Cancer Center
Professor of Medicine and Chief, Nutrition Division
New York Hospital-Cornell Medical Center

Louise B. Russell, Ph.D.
Senior Fellow, Economic Studies Program
The Brookings Institution

Daniel D. Savage, M.D., Ph.D.
Medical Advisor
National Center for Health Statistics
Department of Health and Human Services

David Siscovick, M.D.
Assistant Professor of Medicine and Clinical
  Assistant Professor of Epidemiology
School of Medicine
University of North Carolina at Chapel Hill

Jane E. Sisk, Ph.D.
Senior Associate
Health Program
Office of Technology Assessment
U.S. Congress

Albert J. Stunkard, M.D.
Professor of Psychiatry
Director, Obesity Research Group
University of Pennsylvania

Ernestine Vanderveen, Ph.D.
Chief, Clinical and Psychosocial Research Branch
National Institute on Alcoholism and Alcohol Abuse
Alcohol, Drug Abuse, and Mental Health Administration
Department of Health and Human Services

Milton C. Weinstein, Ph.D.
Henry J. Kaiser Professor of Health Policy and Management
School of Public Health
Harvard University

Brian T. Yates, Ph.D.
Associate Professor
Department of Psychology
The American University

Index

Social Security Amendments of 1983:
  retirement age raised by, 2
Special education: part of
  cost-effectiveness analysis, 73
Spine problems, 49
Stanford Heart Disease Program, 43
Stason, William B., 4, 11–18, 20, 27–28
Stroke: benefit of treatment, 16; cost of
  prevention, 12; and hypertension, 24;
  incidence, 5; as major problem, 67, 23
Stunkard, Albert J., 65, 66
Suicides: and drinking, 57
Surgery: for obesity, 64; among
  smokers, 35
Symptom/problem complexes, 26

Teenage women: calcium intake of, 50
Thiamine deficiency: and alcoholism, 56

United States, alcohol consumption in,
  55; alcoholics in, 56; obesity in, 64
Uric acid, 65

Vaillant, George, 58
Vanderveen, Ernestine, 59–60
Vertebral fractures, 48–49
Veterans' Administration: hypertension
  studies, 11, 13

Weight gain: and osteoporosis, 50
Weight loss: competition, 65; and
  hypertension, 17; over time, 65;
  relation to health, 65
Weight tables: 61
Weight-bearing exercise: and calcium,
  50
Weinstein, Milton C., 4, 11–13, 14–16,
  17–18, 20, 27–28
Well years: state of health measurement
  device, 14, 26–27, 47, 68
Wisconsin: drinking age and accidents
  in, 59
Women: calcium intake of, 50; cancer
  and obesity in, 63; death rate for
  smokers, 34; as drinkers, 55; and
  hypertension, 15–16; increase in
  smoking among, 37; and osteoporosis.
  See Osteoporosis
Work capacity: and disease link, 19–29,
  43
Workers: and smoking, 35–36. See also
  smokers; and Smoking
Wrist fractures, 48

Yano study: osteoporosis, 51
Yates, Brian T., 67
Year of healthy life, 14